COMMUNITY IDEAS FOR IMPROVING THE RESPONSE TO THE DOMESTIC HIV EPIDEMIC

A Report on a National Dialogue on HIV/AIDS

WHITE HOUSE OFFICE OF NATIONAL AIDS POLICY

We thank the following individuals for contributing photographs for this report:

Larry Bryant, Anthony Clark, Anselmo Fonseca, Samuel Johnson, Robert Kohmescher, Sofia Lee, Katrina Lewis, Roy Nelson, Daniel Sampson, Char Smullyan, Steven Underhill

This document was released April 2010 and is available at www.whitehouse.gov/onap.

Acknowledgments

The Office of National AIDS Policy (ONAP) thanks the moderators that facilitated the community discussions, and is grateful for the participation of many community-based organizations, business representatives, and advocates who contributed in immeasurable ways to make these discussions a success. ONAP also gives special thanks to the many people living with or affected by HIV for their courageous and frank testimony that makes this report a compelling and useful document. ONAP also thanks Capital Meeting Planning, Inc., and Impact Marketing for their contributions to the community discussions and to this report; and the State and local elected officials who participated in the community discussions, as well as the following members of Congress:

Senator Al Franken, Minnesota

Delegate Donna M. Christensen, U.S. Virgin Islands

Representative Keith Ellison, Minnesota (5th District)

Representative Eliot Engel, New York (17th District)

Delegate Eleanor Holmes Norton, District of Columbia

Representative Sheila Jackson Lee, Texas (18th District)

Representative Barbara Lee, California (9th District)

Representative John Lewis, Georgia (5th District)

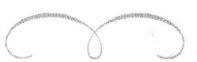

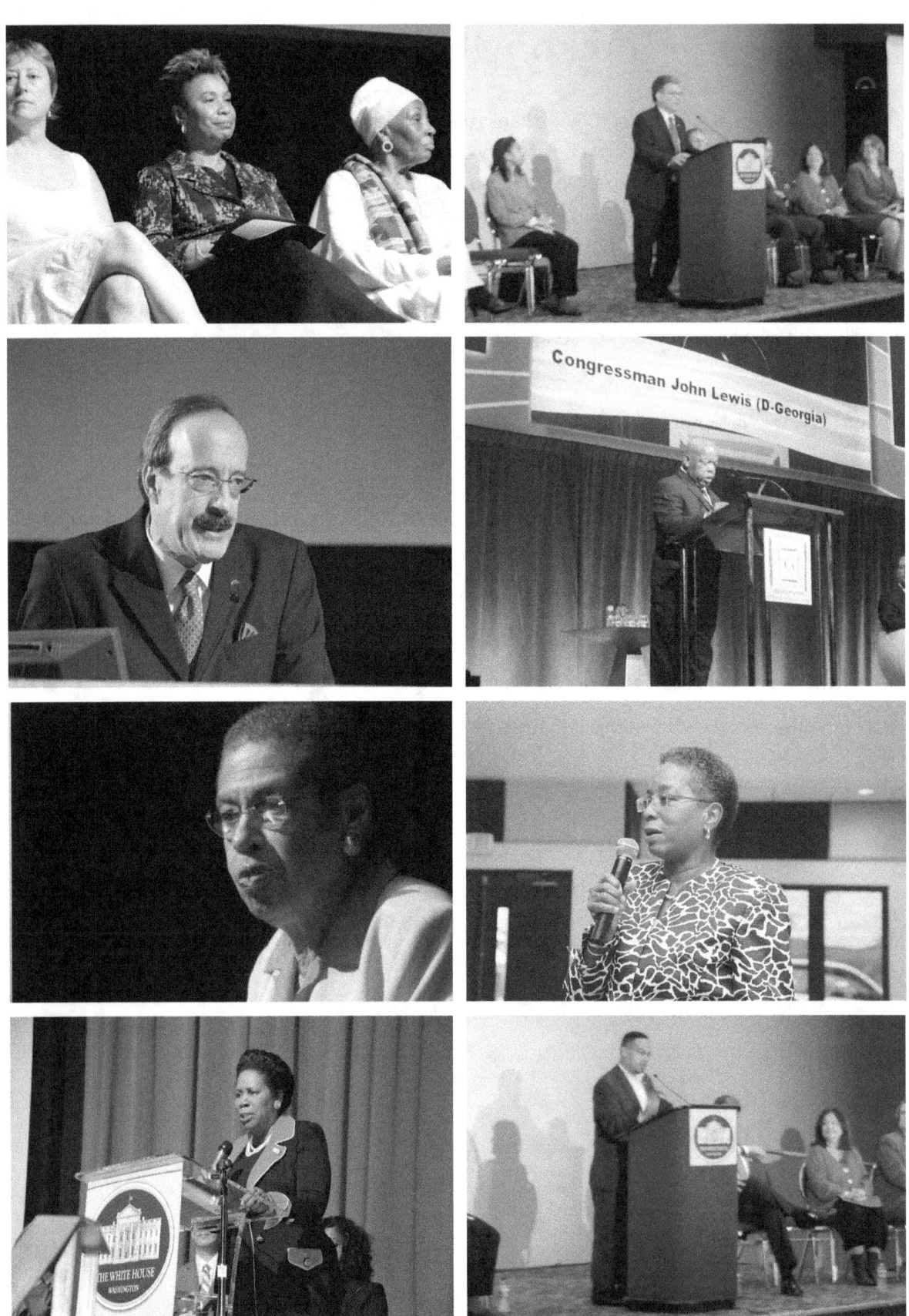

Each member of Congress pictured above attended a community discussion. From the top left to right: Rep. Lee, Sen. Franken, Rep. Engel, Rep. Lewis, Del. Norton, Del. Christensen, Rep. Jackson Lee, Rep. Ellison.

Executive Summary

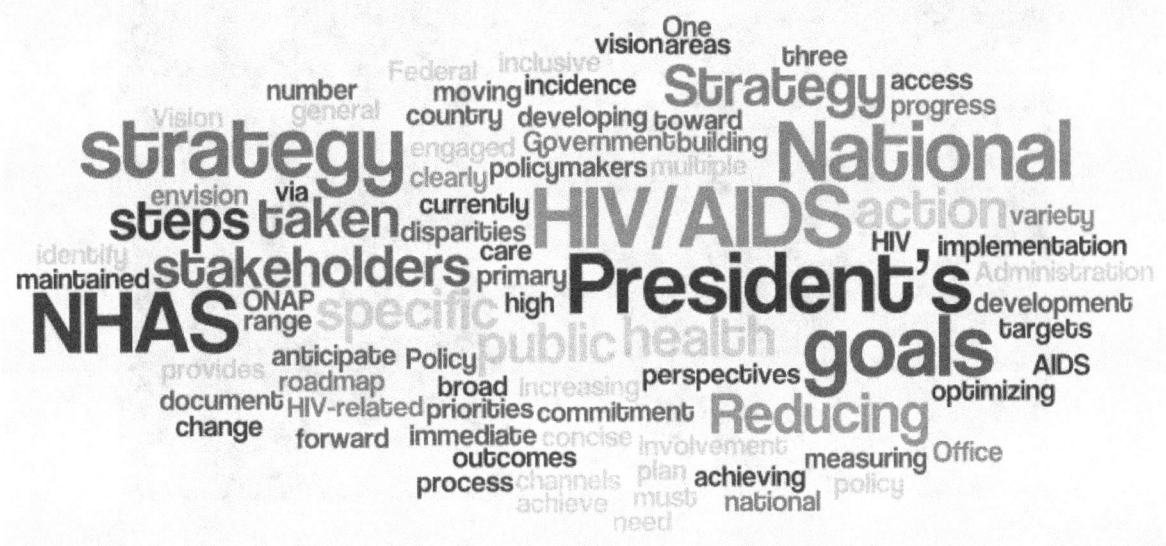

At the beginning of his Administration, President Obama instructed the White House Office of National AIDS Policy (ONAP), a component of the Domestic Policy Council (DPC), to develop a National HIV/AIDS Strategy and re-focus our response to the HIV epidemic in the United States. The President directed that this strategy be driven by three primary goals:

1. Prevent new HIV infections.
2. Increase access to care and optimize health outcomes.
3. Reduce HIV-related health disparities.

From the beginning, ONAP recognized that community involvement was essential in creating a more effective strategy for combating HIV/AIDS in America. To achieve this undertaking, ONAP developed a comprehensive approach for gathering public input and ensuring that ideas from individuals living with HIV, as well as other stakeholders and interested parties, were reflected in the Nation's roadmap for moving forward. ONAP conducted 14 community discussions in locations across the United States and its territories and spoke with more than 4,200 people. ONAP also solicited recommendations for the strategy through the White House Web site. Over 1,000 written recommendations for the National HIV/AIDS Strategy were submitted to ONAP from the community discussions or Web-related submissions. This report is a summary of these community recommendations.

Recommendations related to prevention were made against a backdrop of growing HIV prevalence in the United States. People commonly suggested that we need a broad-based, public information campaign. Individuals told us that this campaign should be vast in scope and should educate a public that remains highly vulnerable to HIV infection. Participants at the community discussions noted that population-specific interventions are crucial. Moreover, they said that any public action must address the numerous social, economic, and behavioral factors that fuel HIV transmission.

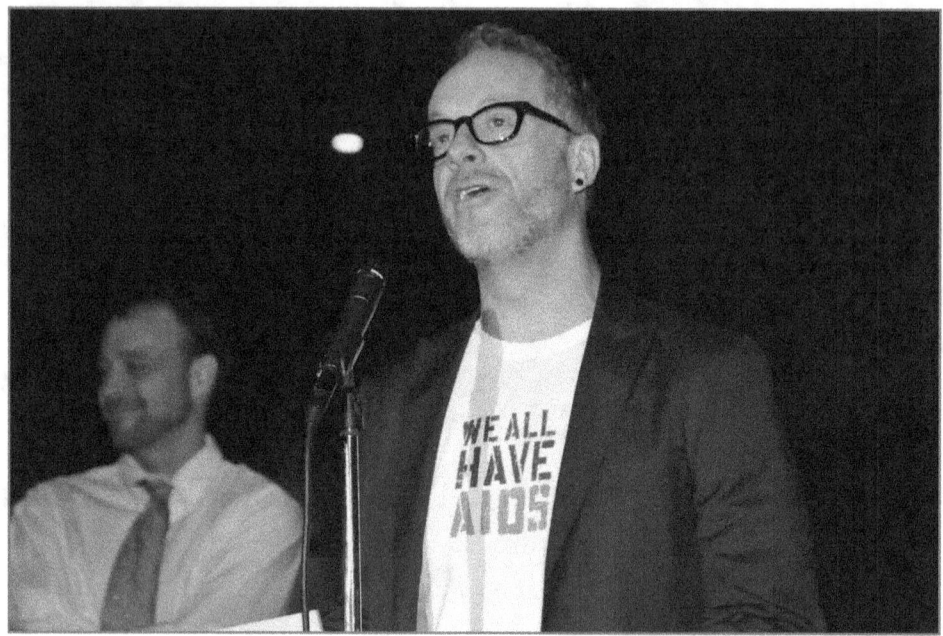

Public comments and written testimonies related to improving access to care shared common themes with those related to prevention and health disparities. In particular, consumers of HIV/AIDS services, as well as services providers and advocates, warned about defining populations too broadly and not recognizing the depth or diversity that exist within subpopulations disproportionately affected by the epidemic. Participants primarily discussed access to care in terms of the broad array of health and social services that are necessary for chronic disease management and long-term wellbeing. They spoke passionately about the need for comprehensive health insurance coverage, culturally competent providers, and a greater number of HIV care providers in underserved rural and urban communities. Perhaps because, comparatively speaking, more people access primary medical care than other services, many testimonies focused on how to make these other services more accessible, including transportation, housing, and job training.

Participants suggested that expanding access to care could help reduce HIV transmission rates and alleviate health disparities. Advocates from or representing vulnerable populations discussed many of the disparities evident in today's epidemic, ranging from racial and ethnic disparities to sex and gender, sexual orientation, age, immigration status, and geographic disparities. Nearly all of the comments referenced the structural inequalities that contribute to these issues. The President's three goals are interconnected, and many participants' recommendations regarding issues, opportunities, and challenges spanned the topics of prevention, access to care, and health disparities. These recommendations most commonly focused on the need for more streamlined funding processes and greater collaboration among Federal, State, and local agencies to facilitate more efficiency. They also addressed the need to increase specificity in the Nation's surveillance data and inequities in the Nation's public and private insurance markets. People also expressed concerns about the shortage of health professionals, specifically of those qualified to address HIV/AIDS, and called for remedies to address this problem.

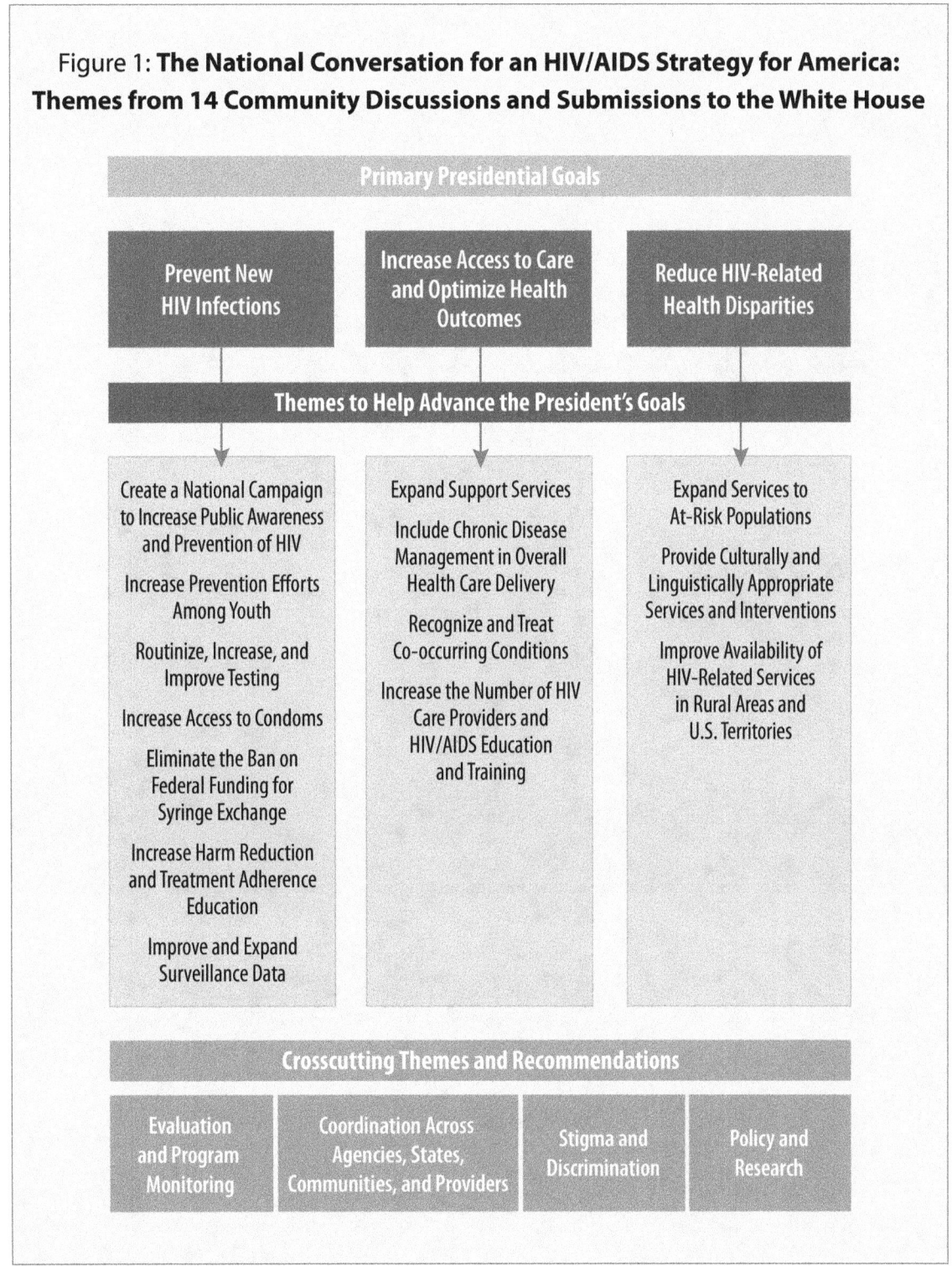

Figure 1: **The National Conversation for an HIV/AIDS Strategy for America: Themes from 14 Community Discussions and Submissions to the White House**

Introduction

"When one of our fellow citizens becomes infected with HIV every nine-and-a-half minutes, the epidemic affects all Americans."

—President Barack Obama

More than 56,000 Americans become infected with HIV each year,[1] and there are more than 1.1 million Americans living with HIV.[2] While infection rates have dropped considerably from previous highs in the 1980s, they have remained flat for many years. HIV is a preventable condition, and every new infection represents a missed opportunity that harms individuals, families, and the Nation as a whole. Although the Nation invests considerable public, private, and personal resources to provide care and support services for people living with HIV, gaps remain. We must do better to bring people into care and ensure they remain within the care system.

This report summarizes a national conversation about HIV/AIDS with the American people. It reflects concerns among Americans from all parts of the country and all socioeconomic backgrounds. It contains a wide range of ideas for addressing the HIV/AIDS epidemic here at home.

The facts driving the need for action are sobering:

- Approximately one in five people living with HIV are unaware that they have HIV, placing them at greater risk for spreading the virus to others.[3]

- Gay and bisexual men and racial/ethnic minorities comprise the greatest proportion of HIV cases in the United States.[4]

- HIV-positive racial and ethnic minorities are more likely to be diagnosed later in their infection and die sooner than Whites.[5]

- One quarter of Americans living with HIV are women, and the disease is disproportionately impacting women of color. HIV/AIDS is one of the leading causes of death among Black women and Latinas.[6]

---

1. CDC. (2009, August). *HIV prevention in the United States at a critical cross roads.* Retrieved from the CDC Web site: http://www.cdc.gov/hiv/resources/reports/hiv_prev_us.htm.
2. CDC. (2008, October 3). HIV Prevalence estimates—United States, 2006. *MMWR, 57(39)*, 1073–1076.
3. CDC. (2008, August). *Estimates of new HIV infections in the United States.* Retrieved from the CDC Web site: http://www.cdc.gov/hiv/topics/surveillance/resources/factsheets/pdf/incidence.pdf., p. 1.
4. CDC. (2009). *HIV/AIDS surveillance report,* 2007, 19, 1–7.
5. CDC. (2009, June 26). Late HIV testing—34 states, 1996-2005. MMWR, 58(24), 661–665.
6. CDC. (2008, August). *HIV/AIDS among Women.* Retrieved from the CDC Web site: http://www.cdc.gov/hiv/topics/women/resources/factsheets/pdf/women.pdf.

- Twenty-nine percent of HIV diagnoses occur among adolescents and young adults (ages 13 to 29).[7]
- Twenty-four percent of people living with HIV are 50 or older, and 15 percent of new HIV/AIDS cases occur among people in this age group.[8]

The President is committed to developing and implementing a National HIV/AIDS Strategy (NHAS) that will focus on reducing HIV incidence, increasing access to care and optimizing health outcomes, and reducing HIV-related health disparities. The NHAS will also increase awareness and promote greater investment in preventing and treating HIV/AIDS in the United States. The White House Office of National AIDS Policy, a component of the Domestic Policy Council, is leading the President's initiative to develop the NHAS.

Because the American people are critical in creating a robust NHAS, ONAP actively and aggressively solicited the best ideas and strategic recommendations from people across the United States.

ONAP heard thousands of Americans' views about the best approaches for addressing HIV/AIDS. We heard from diverse demographic groups and a wide range of ages, income brackets, sexual orientations, education levels, and occupations. Recommendations for the NHAS came from locations as diverse as Minneapolis, San Francisco, Jackson, Mississippi, the U.S. Virgin Islands, and Albuquerque, New Mexico. They came from diverse racial, ethnic, and faith communities and from rural areas, small towns, and large cities. And ONAP listened.

Participants in our national conversation about HIV/AIDS devoted significant attention to this public health crisis and invested a great deal of time crafting public testimony and writing recommendations. Community members presented thoughtful testimony that drew from real life experiences. Their recommendations and personal stories are embodied in this report. They are invaluable tools as ONAP and the Administration work toward drafting an effective strategy that addresses HIV/AIDS in America.

This report summarizes and organizes oral testimony, as well as written and Web-based submissions, in categories that reflect the President's three goals. It also highlights overarching and crosscutting issues related to funding, evaluation, and program integration.

The NHAS will likely identify a small number of targeted, high-payoff actions that can be taken to achieve the President's goals. The Strategy is not intended to be a comprehensive list of all of the actions, policies, and programmatic priorities needed to respond to the domestic HIV epidemic. Rather, it is intended to build upon ongoing public and private initiatives, determine areas where targeted attention can produce results, and identify programs that may benefit from better inter-agency coordination.

---

7. CDC. (2009, August). *HIV/AIDS in the United States*. Retrieved from the CDC Web site: http://www.cdc.gov/hiv/resources/factsheets/PDF/us.pdf., p. 2.

8. CDC. (2008, February). *HIV/AIDS among persons aged 50 and older*. Retrieved from the CDC Web site: http://www.cdc.gov/hiv/topics/over50/resources/factsheets/pdf/over50.pdf., p. 1.

Methodology

From the outset, achieving public input and counsel has been critical to ONAP's approach to creating an NHAS. To foster participation from as many perspectives as possible, ONAP created three mechanisms through which people's voices could be heard: (1) community discussions, (2) written submissions and, (3) online/email submissions to the White House Web site. Each of these mechanisms is described below.

Community Discussions

ONAP conducted 14 community forums and invited the public to discuss its concerns, recommendations, and ideas. The locations for these forums were geographically and demographically diverse. The purpose of these discussions was to hear the unique challenges affecting both large and small communities, and to facilitate meaningful dialogue and recommendations. The community discussions were not designed to be a scientific research study with formal, structured data collection methods.

Diversity in Geography, Diversity in Needs

Many common themes emerged across all community discussions, yet each location highlighted some unique issues to its location:

- In Jackson, Mississippi, the unmet need for transportation services in this predominantly rural State was given significant attention.
- In San Francisco, California, the need for affordable housing in one of the Nation's most-costly housing markets was strongly emphasized.
- In New York City, New York, discussions highlighted growing disparities among infection rates in boroughs like Brooklyn and the Bronx.
- In Albuquerque, New Mexico, there were many Native Americans present while in Oakland, California, participants were predominantly African-American and Latino.
- HIV infection among immigrant communities was a common theme among Africans in Minneapolis and Latinos in Los Angeles.

Community discussions were hosted in the following cities: Atlanta, Georgia; Washington, D.C.; Minneapolis, Minnesota; Albuquerque, New Mexico; Houston, Texas; San Francisco, Los Angeles, and Oakland, California; Columbia, South Carolina; Jackson, Mississippi; Fort Lauderdale, Florida; New York City, New York; Puerto Rico; and the U.S. Virgin Islands. (See Figure 2.) Over 4200 individuals attended the discussions.

Local planning groups comprising State health organizations and local community-based organizations assisted with locating venues and moderators and developing the format of discussions. The meetings were advertised in the communities in which they were held in a variety of ways. The White House issued press releases for each of the meetings, and President Obama referenced the discussions in various speeches, including his speech at the bill signing for the reauthorization of the Ryan White Program.

Moreover, to encourage participation from all members of the community, most discussions provided translation services that included American Sign Language interpretation and Spanish-language translation. Each location was also accessible by public transportation and in compliance with the Americans with Disabilities Act (ADA).

Each of the 14 community discussions was scheduled to last two hours; however, some discussions lasted longer. In an effort to hear as many participants as possible, people were invited to provide remarks for one-and-a-half to two minutes. The specific time allotment depended on the audience size and was established during the ground rules at the beginning of each discussion.

The intent of the community discussions was to collect input for the NHAS and to serve as a vehicle for community members to gather, listen, and share their ideas and experiences. The community discussions were video recorded and uploaded onto the White House Web site.

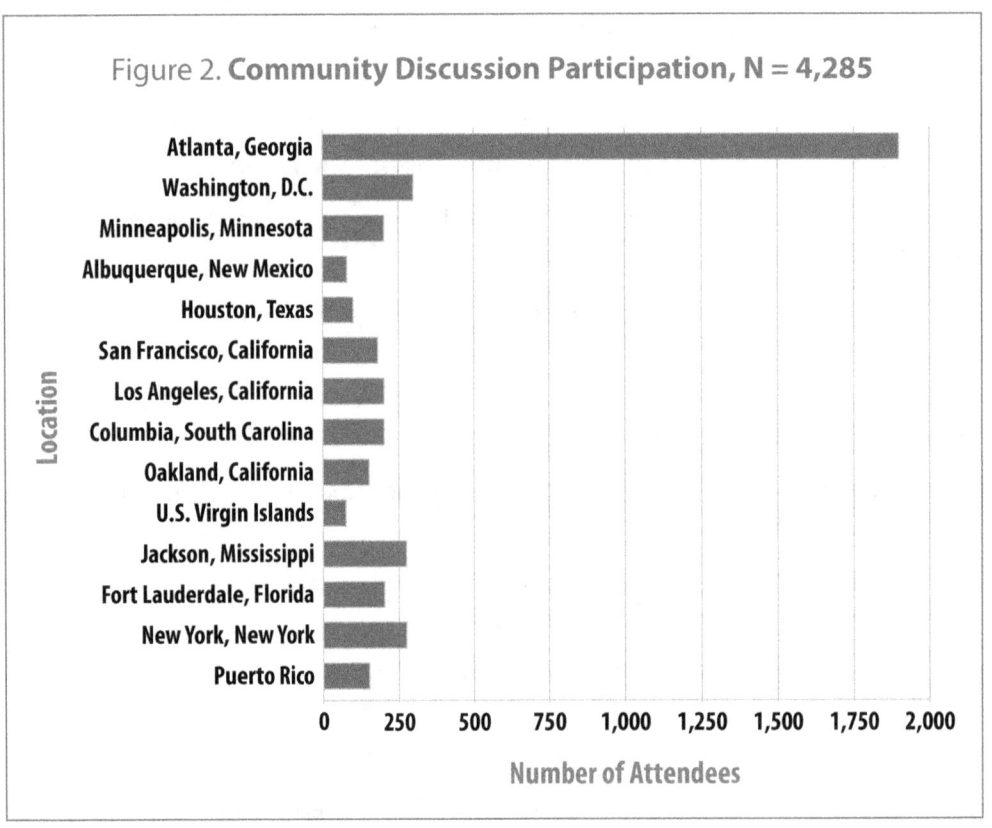

Note: The Atlanta Community Discussion took place during CDC's 2009 National HIV Prevention conference, which had several thousand attendees.

Written Submissions

Individuals who spoke at the community discussions were also encouraged to submit hard copies of their prepared remarks. This gave people an opportunity to provide more comprehensive and detailed suggestions than the oral comment period may have allowed. In many instances, advocacy organizations created and distributed worksheets before the discussion to assist participants in organizing and presenting their input in order to maximize their limited time at the microphone. ONAP received a total of 267 hard-copy written submissions.

Web Submissions

ONAP created a Web-submission mechanism entitled "Call to Action: Americans Speak about HIV/AIDS" that was housed on the ONAP page located on the White House Web site. This allowed ONAP to receive input from individuals across the country regardless of their proximity to the 14 community discussions. The online "Call to Action" also facilitated submissions from people who may have been unwilling or unable to present their comments and recommendations during the community discussions. To maximize participation, the "Call to Action" was included in White House press releases, advertised on various Federal Web sites and listservs, and announced on membership lists of various community advocacy organizations and coalitions.

Individuals were encouraged to complete specific information before they could submit their recommendations to the White House Web site. This included their State or Territory, and affiliation (individual, community-based organization, health care/medical organization, research entity, or State/Federal agency; See Figure 3). Recommendations could be typed directly into a field that accepted 5,000 characters or uploaded as a word processing or PDF file. Because it was not always possible to hear from all participants at the community discussions, participants at the community meetings were encouraged to use the Web-submission mechanism to provide additional recommendations. The "Call to Action" submission process lasted from October 2, 2009, through November 23, 2009, but additional submissions were accepted until early December via the ONAP email address. We received more than 700 Web submissions from 46 States, 3 U.S. territories, and the District of Columbia (See Figure 4.)

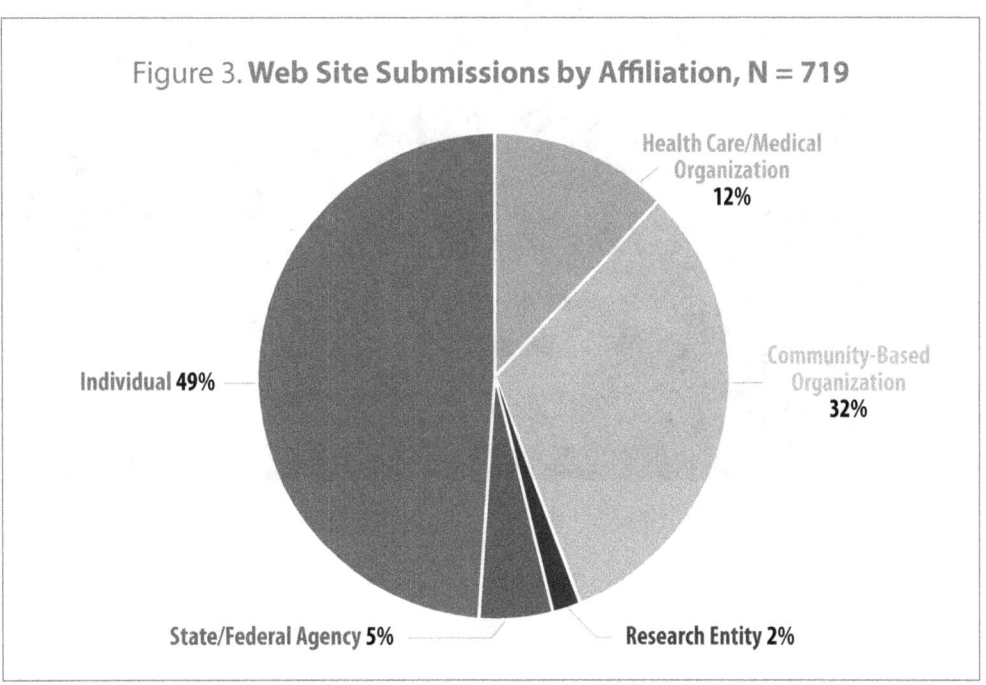

Other Email Submissions

An additional 103 individuals or organizations bypassed the "Call to Action" and submitted recommendations directly to ONAP's email or provided hard-copy recommendations from community-initiated meetings. In some instances, these recommendations were from organizations that submitted more than one document or a particular document with a long list of signatories.

Organizing the Material

A total of 1089* written submissions were received from the community discussions, and from email, Web, and hard-copy submissions. These submissions were integrated into a single list to organize and highlight key findings across communities. ONAP reviewed and organized all of the recommendations put forward for consideration. An outline of major topic areas was created after reading through the material and for the purposes of organizing this report.

Submissions have been organized and discussed in this report with the objective of providing a comprehensive written record and creating a planning tool for the NHAS development process.

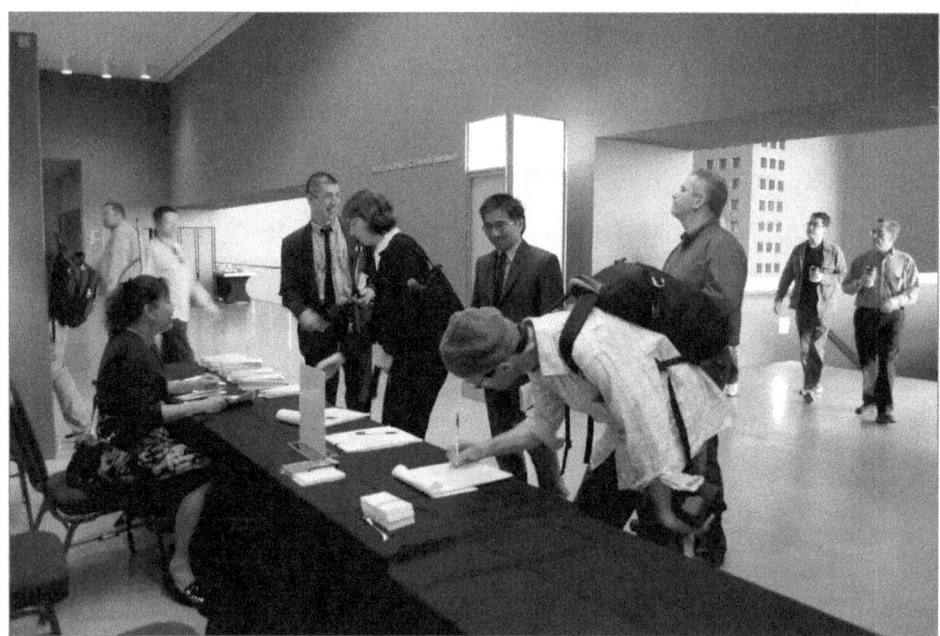

---

* Tallies were created from counting individual comments or group submissions where possible; those numbers are reflected in the tables and charts in this chapter. Please note these numbers are approximate. In cases where identical recommendations were submitted through multiple channels, those recommendations were counted only once and through the channel from which they were first received

METHODOLOGY

Figure 4. **Web site Submissions by State/U.S. Territory, N=719**

Alabama	7	Hawaii	3	Mississippi	9	Rhode Island	4
Alaska	3	Idaho	1	Missouri	8	Puerto Rico	9
American Samoa	1	Illinois	22	Nevada	2	South Carolina	13
Arizona	9	Indiana	7	Nebraska	2	Tennessee	9
Arkansas	9	Iowa	6	New Hampshire	2	Texas	23
California	102	Kansas	3	New Jersey	8	Vermont	1
Colorado	6	Kentucky	7	New Mexico	12	Virginia	14
Connecticut	7	Louisiana	20	New York	109	Virgin Islands	6
Delaware	1	Maine	2	North Carolina	10	Washington	21
District of Columbia	19	Maryland	13	Ohio	26	West Virginia	4
Florida	56	Massachusetts	16	Oklahoma	7	Wisconsin	2
Georgia	22	Michigan	6	Oregon	13		
Guam	1	Minnesota	22	Pennsylvania	34		

+No Web-based submissions were received from individuals or organizations in Montana, North Dakota, South Dakota, Utah, Wyoming, or the U.S. Territory Northern Mariana Islands.

■ Blue indicates a State or territory where comments have been received.

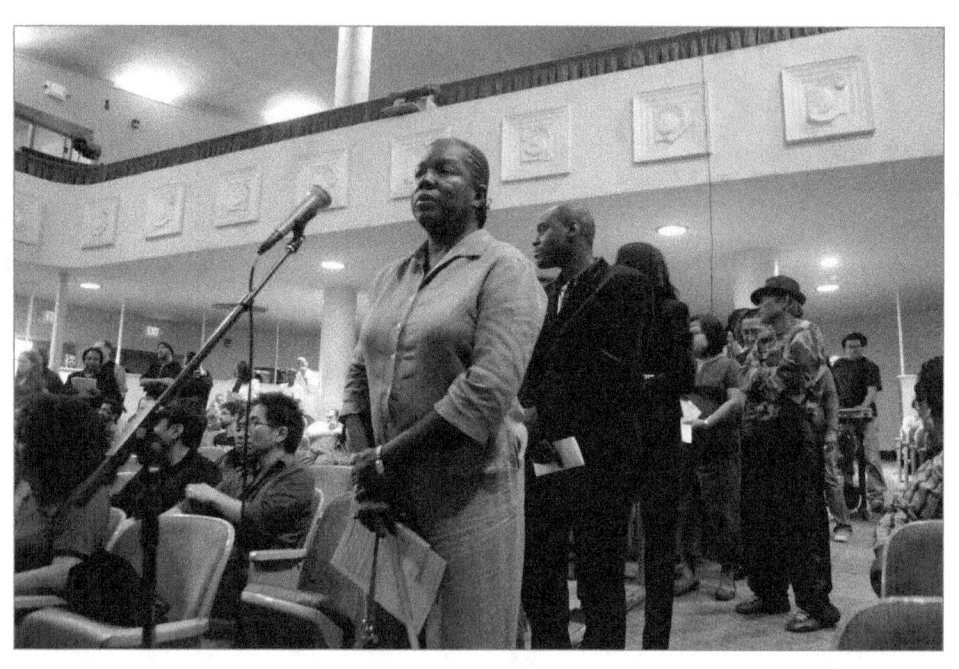
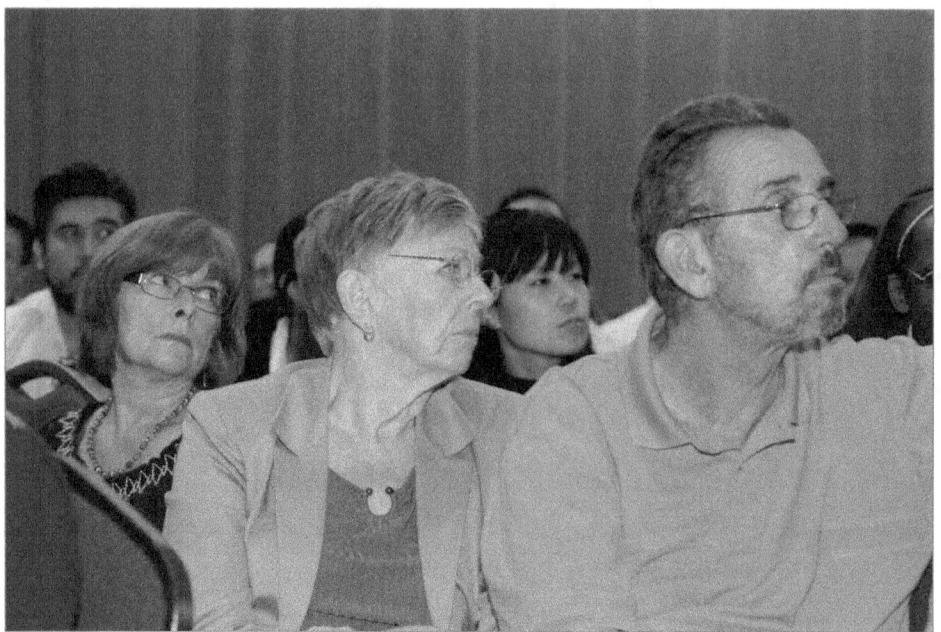

Preventing HIV Transmission

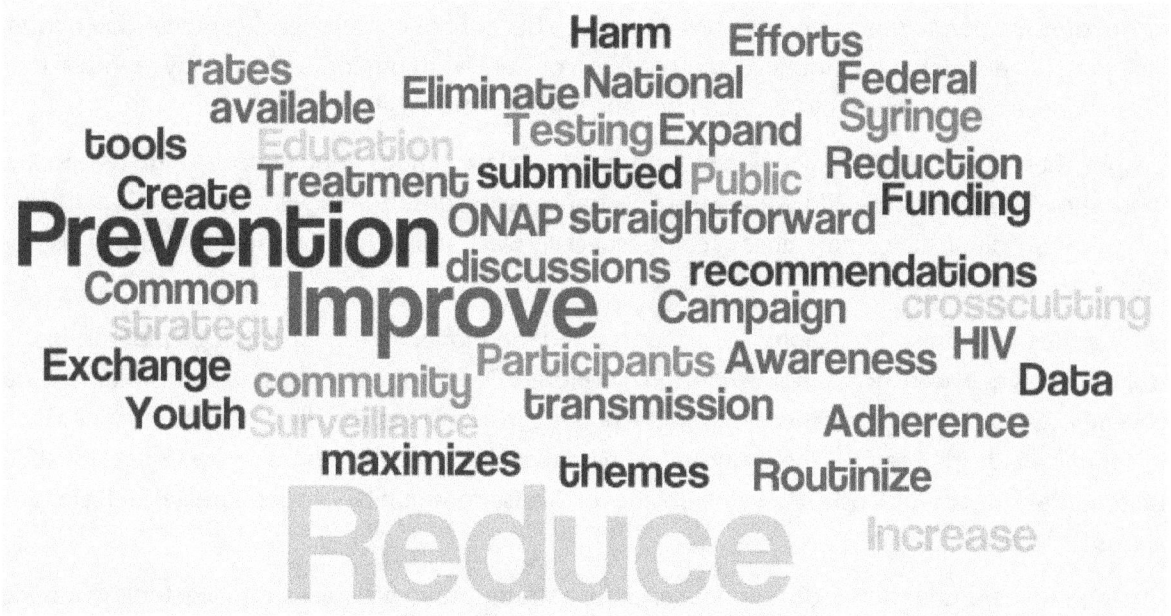

The first cases of what later became known as AIDS were reported in June of 1981.[9] Otherwise healthy men were diagnosed with rare infections including Pneumocystis pneumonia—a disease seen only in immunosuppressed patients.[10] By 1990, more than 100,000 individuals had died of AIDS.[11]

We have come a long way since the beginning of the epidemic and, thankfully, there have been many successes in preventing HIV since the 1980s. The Centers for Disease Control and Prevention (CDC) has reported that the number of new infections dropped from more than 130,000 per year in the mid-1980s to just over 56,000 per year by 2006.[12,13] In 1994, findings from the Pediatric AIDS Clinical Trial Group 076 showed that an AZT (Zidovudine) regimen reduced perinatal transmission of HIV by two-thirds.[14] AZT was quickly recommended for use in all HIV-positive pregnant women, and mother-to-child transmission plummeted. Today, with proper treatment throughout pregnancy, perinatal HIV transmission cases have declined.[15]

---

9. CDC. (2006, June 2). Epidemiology of HIV/AIDS—United States, 1981-2005. MMWR, 55(21), 589–592.

10. CDC. (1981, June 5). Pneumocystis pneumonia—Los Angeles. MMWR, 30(21), 1–3.

11. CDC. *Current Trends in Mortality Attributable to HIV Infection/AIDS United States, 1981–1990*. January 1991: 41–44.

12. CDC. (2008, August). *Estimates of new HIV infections in the United States*. Retrieved from the CDC Web site: http://www.cdc.gov/nchhstp/Newsroom/docs/Fact-Sheet-on-HIV-Estimates.pdf., p. 2.

13. CDC. (2009, August). *HIV prevention in the United States at a critical cross roads*. Retrieved from the CDC Web site: http://www.cdc.gov/hiv/resources/reports/hiv_prev_us.htm.

14. Connor, E.M., Sperling, R.S., Gelber, R., Kiselev, P., Scott, G., O'Sullivan, M.J.,& Balsley, J. (1994, November 3). Reduction of maternal-infant transmission of human immunodeficiency virus type 1 with zidovudine treatment. *New England Journal of Medicine*, 18(331), 1173–1180.

15. CDC. (2007, October). *Mother-to-child (perinatal) HIV transmission and prevention*. Retrieved from the CDC Web site: http://www.cdc.gov/hiv/topics/perinatal/resources/factsheets/perinatal.htm., p. 3.

In 1995, combination therapy, also known as highly active antiretroviral therapy (HAART), was introduced.[16,17,18] HAART dramatically increased survival rates and improved quality of life for people living with HIV, while also reducing infectiousness among people living with HIV and the probability of HIV transmission to uninfected persons. Moreover, because of comprehensive prevention efforts, including needle exchange programs and provision of sterile equipment, CDC recently reported that HIV incidence has decreased by 80 percent among injection drug users.[19]

Despite these successes, the HIV epidemic continues to place various populations at high risk. Today, men who have sex with men (MSM), are the only transmission group where HIV incidence is markedly increasing. Additionally, communities of color, especially Black and Latino communities, remain disproportionately affected by HIV.

During the community discussions, participants often mentioned that the HIV/AIDS epidemic in the United States has been increasingly forgotten or ignored. Despite the diminishing mainstream media coverage, and a shrinking presence of HIV in the public consciousness, the HIV epidemic remains a reality for many individuals across the country. We heard that HIV prevention in the United States must be bold, address the complex risks and vulnerabilities of diverse communities, and streamline inefficiencies across Federal agencies.

Participants in the community discussions called for a strategy that maximizes available tools to reduce transmission rates. The recommendations submitted to ONAP were straightforward and often crosscutting. Common themes that we heard include:

A. Create a National Campaign to Increase Public Awareness and Prevention of HIV

"...a national social marketing campaign that states the facts about condoms and their ability to prevent HIV just like the seatbelt campaign that we all saw in the 1980s."

—Houston, Texas community discussion

There is a lack of knowledge related to HIV risk and transmission across broad segments of the American public. "I hear from middle and high school students that having or living with STDs is just the way it is going to be....There is a lot of misconceptions in the media that is leading them to believe it is no big

---

16. HAART refers to a pharmaceutical regimen that involves taking a combination of antiretroviral medications. Initial HAART therapies included at least one protease inhibitor, but new treatment combinations exist that do not contain protease inhibitors.

17. Baker R. (1995, December). FDA approves 3TC and saquinavir. San Francisco AIDS Foundation. *Bulletin of Experimental Treatments for AIDS.* 5–9.

18. KFF. (2007, December). *Global HIV/AIDS timelines*. Retrieved from the KFF Web site: http://www.kff.org/hivaids/timeline/hivtimeline.cfm.

19. CDC. (2008, August). *Estimates of new HIV infections in the United States*. Retrieved from the CDC Web site: http://www.cdc.gov/nchhstp/Newsroom/docs/Fact-Sheet-on-HIV-Estimates.pdf., p. 2.

deal," explained an AIDS activist in New Mexico. The absence of information related to HIV/AIDS, and only a partial understanding of HIV risk, is fueling new infections in the United States every year.

The participants called for a far-reaching, more comprehensive approach to increasing public awareness about HIV/AIDS.

Audiences

"[Our] interactions with other AIDS service organizations keeps awareness of HIV high [among our congregants]…so we can continue to be on the forefront of responding…and ministering to those whom it affects."

—Episcopal Church representative Web submission

Participants in public forums across the country emphasized that a single message and approach will not evoke the desired response among all target audiences. "Begin a coordinated education campaign with identified individuals…and definitely connect to the African-American community," recommended one participant. "People seem to have forgotten middle-class White women who have been divorced recently, and who do not have a clue that HIV exists. Education needs to be given to them too," added another.

The target audiences for a national campaign must be segmented to reflect population-specific barriers to information and behavior change. "I am an Asian Pacific Islander transgender woman. I face different issues than my gay brothers, and I have different needs," explained one respondent.

Many participants suggested that culturally-appropriate messages and message delivery strategies be crafted to address diverse populations. They recommended that unique messaging, messengers, and delivery mechanisms be developed for audiences defined by the following characteristics:

- **Risk category.** Participants requested messaging that addresses the risks of specific communities.
- **Age.** These messages should be unique and crafted for specific age brackets, beginning with youth still in school and ranging to older adults. Participants noted the need to reach people early in life, and to continue to tailor risk reduction messages for individuals as they age. Several participants highlighted the need to address HIV prevention messages for people over the age of 50, as well as HIV care services for people living with HIV as they age or those who seroconvert as seniors.
- **Race/ethnicity.** Participants said that these messages should also be crafted for the five racial categories currently tracked in CDC surveillance reports (White, Black, Latino, Asian/ Pacific Islander, American Indian/Alaska Native) and for other racial and ethnic populations as well, such as Arab Americans and Africans who have recently immigrated to America.
- **Gender.** In addition to establishing culturally-appropriate approaches to target males and females, participants also voiced how important it is to craft a national HIV education campaign targeting transgender individuals, many of whom are not reached by current messaging.

Messages, Messengers, and Message Placement

"Effective health education and HIV/AIDS prevention education has been proven to work when methods are used that are science and research based."
—Los Angeles, California community discussion

Many participants called for science-driven prevention messages. They urged that information regarding issues like safer sex and risk reduction be defined by scientifically-proven—rather than ideologically-driven—approaches to reducing HIV incidence.

However, even the best messages are only as effective as the messenger. Participants suggested that potential messengers include:

- Peers within each of the risk behavior groups,
- Peers from LGBTQ communities,
- Key influencers with whom at-risk groups identify, including parents, teachers, faith-based leaders, and community leaders, and
- Opinion leaders, such as political and other publicly recognized officials.

Many of the comments advocated for enlisting trusted community leaders and stakeholders to help engage community members and spotlight public health needs. "Bring education to Native Tribes and Native American community-based organizations and get buy-in from leaders," suggested one Albuquerque man. Take "our hip hop community and utilize it to disseminate information to the people who are most prevalent in catching [HIV] disease," recommended a Houston resident.

"There is no education in our tribes," said an Albuquerque man. Stressing the need for culturally-specific efforts, he explained, "There are over 300 tribes or nations…We are different people. I myself am an Apache, [and] cannot speak up [for] a Pueblo or a Navajo here in New Mexico. [We] have different ways."

The difficulty of reaching out to young people was emphasized repeatedly, with many participants urging parents and schools to become actively involved in delivering risk-reduction messages to youth. There was widespread support for providing information about male and female condoms to audiences of all ages.

The need to embed HIV prevention within a cultural context was repeatedly noted at locations across the country. As one San Francisco resident explained,

"A/PI's [Asian and Pacific Islanders] are not one ethnic or racial group. They are 40 different ethnicities speaking over 100 different languages. As long as they do not see pictures of people living with HIV who are also A/PIs, they will never realize that HIV is something that will affect their community adversely."

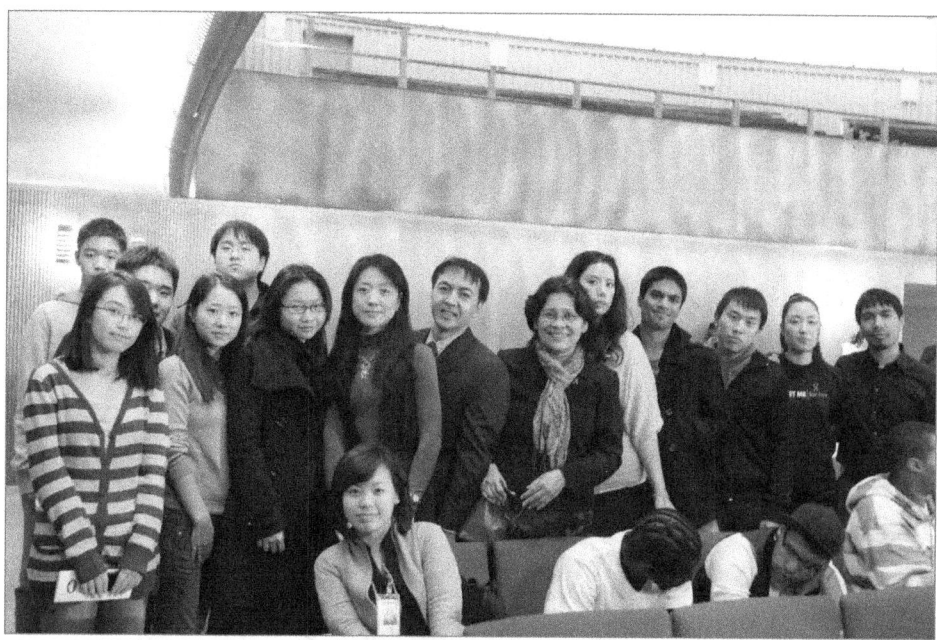

Participants also highlighted the importance of distributing risk-reduction information in specific locations, such as schools, faith-based institutions, and social-services organizations. HIV prevention efforts should be visible wherever people at high risk for infection can be found. "Women that are incarcerated both in jails and prisons need this information," stated a Jackson, Mississippi resident.

Respondents urged broader use of print, radio, mail, and, especially, television in a more widespread and far-reaching campaign. "Do what Surgeon General Koop did in 1988 and mail each U.S. household an updated brochure on HIV/AIDS and include current trends, statistics, myth busters, HIV prevention and treatment information, and information to online resources," suggested a Sacramento, California woman. A more public and more visible platform for HIV prevention efforts was also discussed. Participants recommended that a national campaign be visible on television and employ new media platforms that harness the power of virtual communities.

B. Increase Prevention Efforts Among Youth

"I am tired of telling teenagers that their HIV test is positive.... Every 17-year-old I diagnose with HIV represents 60 to 80 years of transmission potential [and] each represents nearly a million dollars in health care costs over their lifetime."

——Minneapolis, Minnesota community discussion

Written submissions and public testimonies across the country highlighted the need for population-specific approaches to HIV prevention and care efforts to reduce health disparities. Participants discussed the unique challenges faced by racial and ethnic minorities, sexual minorities, and women. They gave significant attention to the needs of young people and emphasized the importance of preventing HIV infections as early as possible.

Participants repeatedly highlighted how critical prevention efforts are among young people. Young people[20] accounted for an estimated 29 percent of new HIV infections in 2006.[21] Youth also represent one of the most medically underserved populations in the United States, and they are often unaware of their HIV status.

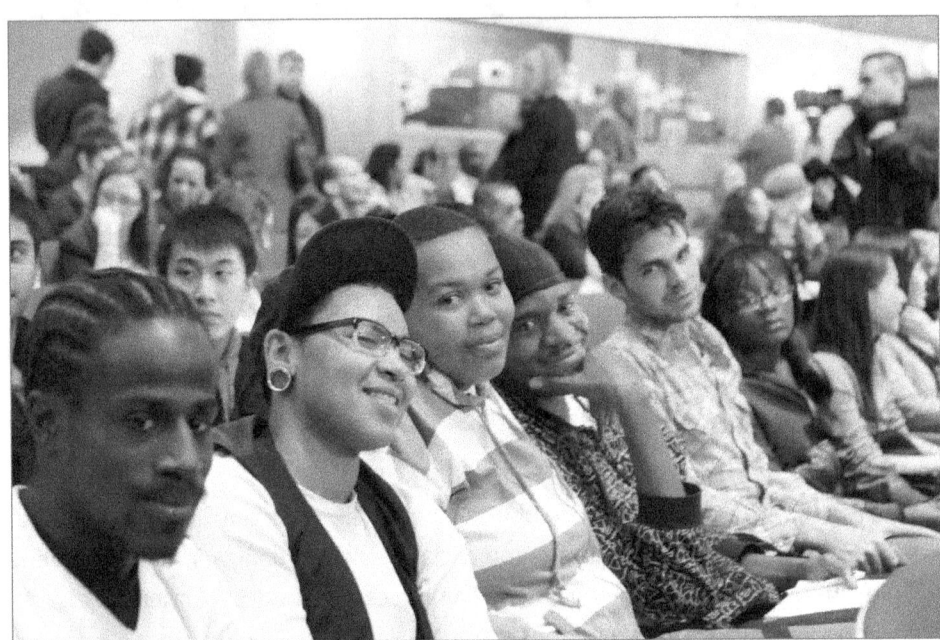

A student in St. Croix wrote, "We need the U.S. Government to keep youth informed on the facts about HIV and AIDS…and to get more serious about our behaviors." The majority of HIV-positive youth become infected through behaviors like drug use or sexual intercourse. Although there are relatively few annual perinatal infections in the United States, we heard from several community members that prevention of perinatal infection should remain a priority. As one participant stressed,

"I was born HIV positive….[at] a time when we did not have medications to prevent mother-to-child transmission….That is not the case anymore. We can prevent it…there is absolutely no reason why more children should be infected and a generation should continue going forward being HIV positive."

Participants discussed the need to reach youth early and often, and called for comprehensive sexuality education to take place both in school settings and in other venues where youth are found. Many advocated that this education be science-based and include information pertinent to all sexual orientations, condom use, and HIV and other STDs. Virtually whenever community members spoke about HIV prevention for young people, they advocated for comprehensive, evidence-based sexuality education.

---

20. In this instance, young people refer to people under the age of 30.
21. CDC. (2009, August). *HIV/AIDS in the United States*. Retrieved from the CDC Web site: www.cdc.gov/hiv/resources/factsheets/PDF/us.pdf., p. 2.

Many people demanded that the Federal Government stop funding abstinence-only education initiatives. As one respondent summarized, "Teach…the benefits of abstinence without demonizing those who are sexually active."

"HIV/AIDS prevention education does not need to be reinvented, but such efforts do need teeth in mandating laws to ensure that programs are really provided by qualified teachers as designed and evaluated to maintain effectiveness," asserted one respondent.

An Albuquerque, New Mexico resident stated, "It is important that our youth get correct and factual messages for them using all types of media and technical methods of communication."

C. Routinize, Increase, and Improve Testing

"The first step toward HIV treatment is getting tested, knowing your status."

—Columbia, South Carolina community discussion

An estimated 21 percent of HIV-positive persons in the United States do not know their status.[22] Besides compromising their long-term health outcomes due to delayed care, undiagnosed individuals may unknowingly place their sexual partners at risk for HIV transmission. According to a CDC study, between 54 to 70 percent of new HIV transmissions in the United States are due to people with unrecognized HIV infection.[23]

Studies indicate that people who are diagnosed with HIV reduce their risk behaviors with HIV-negative partners to minimize the possibility of transmission.[24] "I have not infected anyone and I am undetectable now," said a California man on the prevention value that HIV-testing has for reinforcing responsible behaviors.

Access to HIV testing should also be expanded to help individuals learn their HIV status earlier in the course of their illness. According to a CDC analysis of 34 States with confidential name-based reporting, 38.3 percent of persons with a new HIV diagnosis developed AIDS within one year.[25] Without treatment, most people live for close to a decade from the time of infection until they are diagnosed with AIDS. This high percentage of people who are diagnosed with AIDS so soon after learning their HIV status suggests that we are not reaching many people until they have been living with HIV for many years. Many factors cause late testing, including underestimating HIV risk. This leads to delayed care, poorer health outcomes, increased morbidity and mortality, and more opportunities for HIV transmission.

---

22. CDC. (2008, October). *New estimates of U.S. HIV prevalence*, 2006. Retrieved from the CDC Web site: http://www.cdc.gov/nchhstp/newsroom/docs/prevalence.pdf., p. 1.

23. Marks, G., Crepaz, N., & Janssen, R. (2006). Estimating sexual transmission of HIV from persons aware and unaware that they are infected with the virus in the USA. *AIDS, 20*(10), 1447–1450.

24. CDC. (2008, August 3). *HIV Testing*. Retrieved from the CDC Web site: http://www.cdc.gov/hiv/topics/testing/.

25. CDC. (2009, June 26). Late HIV testing—34 states, 1996-2005. *MMWR, 58(24)*, 661–665.

Participant recommendations related to HIV testing largely fall into four categories:

- Routinize HIV testing.
- Encourage HIV testing.
- Locate HIV testing in nontraditional settings.
- Improve the content of the testing encounter.

Routinize HIV Testing

To increase overall testing, diagnose HIV infection early, and engage HIV-positive persons in appropriate medical treatment, CDC recently revised its testing recommendations to include routine screenings of 13- to 64-year-olds in health care settings.

(To learn more, visit http://www.cdc.gov/hiv/topics/testing/healthcare/index.htm.) In short, CDC recommends that all adults and adolescents get tested for HIV as part of their regular medical care.

Community discussion participants emphasized putting existing CDC guidelines into practice. "I'd recommend providing adequate funding for implementing the CDC guidelines and making this approach a program of national priority just like the prevention of perinatal transmission in the late 1990s," suggested one Web respondent who was referencing the AIDS Clinical Trial Group 076 that proved perinatal transmission could be cut dramatically.

Participants also stated that testing should continue to be accompanied with referrals and counseling, and that the government should assist organizations in expanding HIV testing. Several participants advocated for co-locating HIV testing in primary care settings to encourage seamless linkage to care. Although some pushed for universal HIV testing, others advocated HIV testing for targeted groups. There was consensus that HIV testing should be voluntary.

Encourage HIV Testing

"Psychological science has shown if we don't talk about it… people feel it must not matter."

—Newburgh, New York Web submission

Participants advised that a population-specific approach be designed to ensure that messages, messengers, and distribution mechanisms reflect the needs and realities of diverse demographic groups. They noted that risk factors are not the only elements that should drive the creation of testing promotion strategies, and they stated other demographic characteristics such as race and gender are also critical.

Participants reminded ONAP that to provide a framework for promoting HIV testing among the general population, stigma must be considered and addressed. They also noted that routinization of HIV testing, coupled with visible involvement and encouragement from well-known individuals, community leaders, and peers, is critical. Public comments also stressed separating HIV testing from other issues, such as immigration and fear of deportation, as well the importance of partner notification.

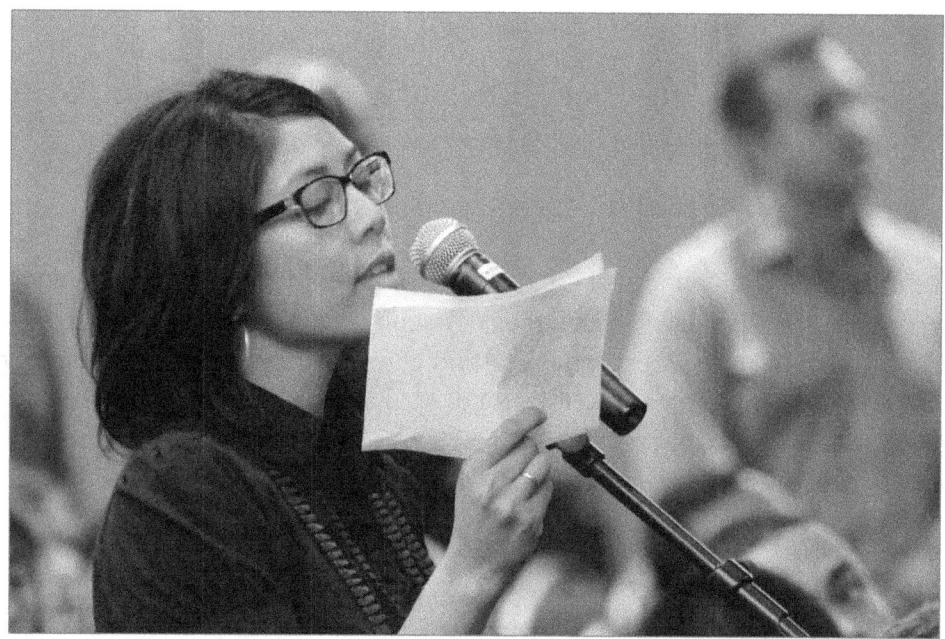

Partner notification involves trained public health specialists locating and contacting any person whose name has been supplied by an HIV-positive partner or his/her health provider. Utilizing partner notification is sometimes the best—and quickest—way to ensure partners are contacted.[26] As one social worker in Minneapolis, Minnesota described, "There needs to be an overhaul of partner notification services nationally to address antiquated and underperforming systems, health campaigns to sell the importance of partner notification services to the public, update training, and incorporate new technologies to more effectively and efficiently notify individuals of their possible exposures…When conducted effectively, partner notification services are a proven method to reduce HIV incidence and increase access to care for those at risk."

Locate HIV Testing in Nontraditional Settings

"People in our community [were] deciding to die rather than get tested—so great was the stigma in some parts of our community."

—Washington, D.C. community discussion

The theme of making testing more widely available was also prevalent in many discussions and submissions. This included a call for continued outreach with mobile vans or peers on foot to find hard-to-reach individuals who are often the last to enter care. Other recommendations included increasing access and reducing the cost barrier to at-home testing devices; making testing more widely available and encouraged in corrections institutions; incorporating testing into dental visits; and allowing testing in nonclinical settings where at-risk populations frequent.

---

26. CDC. (2007, August 16). *Program operations guidelines for STD prevention: partner services*. Retrieved from the CDC Web site: http://www.cdc.gov/STD/Program/partner/6-PGpartner.htm.

Improve the Content of the HIV Testing Encounter

"Geriatric specialists must include HIV testing as a routine test…Taboos in this generation, such as not speaking about sex, have to be addressed diligently."

—San Juan, Puerto Rico Web submission

Comments suggested the importance of using every encounter to provide as much information and support as possible. There is a divide within the community over whether we need to re-emphasize pre- and post-test counseling as we expand HIV testing or whether this serves as a barrier to expanded testing, or even whether this stigmatizes HIV testing. Many participants noted that some individuals who test for HIV never return for test results. Participants also discussed the need to provide negotiating skills for individuals at risk for contracting HIV/AIDS.

D. Increase Access to Condoms

"[T]he effect of Black American heterosexual men who do not use condoms and engage in concurrent relationships or have multiple sex partners, plays a most significant role in the exposure of Black American women."

—Oakland, California community discussion

Sexual Transmission of HIV

Eighty-five percent of new infections result from sexual transmission.

Men who have sex with men (MSM), account for an estimated 4 percent of the male population in the United States, but 53 percent of all new HIV infections, making them both the single largest risk group and the group most disproportionately at risk for HIV infection.

MSM are more than 44–86 times more likely to become infected than other men in the United States, and 40–77 times more likely to become infected compared to women. Within this at-risk population, Black and Latino MSM are more likely than Whites to become infected with HIV.

Among the 26 percent of cases among women, Black women account for an estimated 60 percent of all new infections. The majority of HIV cases among women are due to sexual behavior with men.

Sources: CDC. (2009, August). *HIV/AIDS in the United States: CDC HIV/AIDS facts*. Retrieved from the CDC Web site: http://www.cdc.gov/hiv/resources/factsheets/PDF/us.pdf. CDC. (2009). *HIV/AIDS Surveillance Report*. 2007,19, Table 3.
CDC. (2010), *CDC Analysis Provides New Look at Disproportionate Impact of HIV and Syphilis Among U.S. Gay and Bisexual Men*. Retrieved from the CDC Web site: http://www.cdc.gov/nchhstp/Newsroom/msmpressrelease.html.

Over 80 percent of new HIV/AIDS diagnoses among adults and adolescents in the United States in 2007 were related to sexual activity.[27] Virtually all of these cases could have been prevented. "The Federal Government needs to sponsor and fund the broad based availability of male and female condoms in HIV and STD impacted communities across America," urged a San Francisco woman representing one of a number of participants calling for increased access to condoms in prevention efforts.

Several individuals recommended expanding access to safer sex materials and needle exchange programs. Many people advocated for the distribution of condoms in schools, as well as in prisons and jails. Several people also stated that we must lower financial barriers to condoms and make them easier to access in pharmacies.

As one participant summarized, "Teaching people how to use condoms is no longer [enough]....They need to have their positive self identity improved so that they feel like they are important and they need to take care of themselves." Building self esteem and increasing access to information about condoms was echoed throughout submissions and community discussions.

E. Eliminate the Ban on Federal Funding for Syringe Exchange

"Understand that syringe exchange is the gateway to treatment and we need to take the obstacles and hurdles out of people getting into [care]."

—Washington, D.C. community discussion

Injection drug use (IDU) accounted for 17 percent of new HIV diagnoses among adults and adolescents diagnosed in 2007.[28] An additional 3 percent of newly diagnosed cases were attributed to MSM/IDU.[29] IDU also accounts for the most hepatitis C (HCV) infections in the United States, and co-infection of HIV/HCV can complicate both treatment and health outcomes.[30]

Research indicates that syringe exchange programs are cost effective and have positive impacts in reducing the spread of HIV. According to a cohort study published in the *Journal of Acquired Immune Deficiency Syndromes*, IDUs involved in syringe-exchange programs are up to six times less likely to put themselves at risk of HIV infection.[31] Access and funding for such programs, however, have been limited by both State laws and a Federal ban on funding for such programs. Many participants recommended eliminating the ban on Federal funding for syringe exchange programs. Another recommendation was to expand access to syringe exchange programs in pharmacies.

---

27. CDC. (August 2009). *HIV/AIDS in the United States*. Retrieved from the CDC Web site: http://www.cdc.gov/hiv/resources/factsheets/PDF/us.pdf., p. 1.

28. Ibid., 1.

29. CDC. (August 2009). *HIV/AIDS in the United States*. Retrieved from the CDC Web site: http://www.cdc.gov/hiv/resources/factsheets/PDF/us.pdf., p. 1.

30. CDC. Hepatitis C information for the public. n.d. Available at: http://www.cdc.gov/hepatitisC/index.htm. Accessed December 3, 2009.

31. Gibson, D.R., Brand, R., Anderson, K., Kahn, J.G., Perales, D., & Guydish, J. (2002, October 1). Two- to six-fold decreased odds of HIV risk behavior associated with use of syringe exchange. *Journal of Acquired Immune Deficiency Syndromes*, 31(2), 237.

In November 2009, Congress lifted the ban on using Federal funding for needle and syringe exchange programs. The lifting of this ban was welcomed by the Administration and seen as another step toward policy informed by science and not ideology.

F. Increase Harm Reduction and Treatment Adherence Education

"We must have more comprehensive harm reduction programs available across the Nation that includes needle exchange."

—Asheville, North Carolina Web submission

Harm Reduction

In the context of HIV prevention, harm reduction commonly refers to minimizing risk associated with one's behavior. This may include condom use, although it often refers to the reduction of drug-related harm, such as syringe exchange programs (described in section E) and medication-assisted drug therapy. A guiding principle of harm reduction interventions is to meet people where they are and to work with them to decrease risk to the fullest extent possible. The phrase "where they are" can refer to individuals and their struggles with addiction or unprotected sexual activity. It also refers to where people are in a literal sense, such as corrections institutions, substance abuse treatment facilities, health clinics, or other key points of entry in the medical system.

"Jails are a perfect opportunity to offer evidence-based prevention interventions ... it is less expensive to be proactive in our prevention efforts [and] to foster behavior change among those at high risk for HIV transmission," expressed a respondent from Wilkinsburg, Pennsylvania, emphasizing the need to intervene among those at highest risk for HIV infection and among those already living with the disease.

Treatment and Adherence

Medical treatment and adherence are two of the many services for people living with HIV that can help reduce HIV transmission. People living with HIV who take antiretroviral therapy have lower viral loads and are less infectious than those not on therapy, and they also have better health-related outcomes.

Many participants discussed the importance of working with people living with HIV to help stop HIV transmission. "Treatment education is a crucial tool for the success of antiretroviral therapy and long-term adherence," stated one Web respondent. These are important components of any strategy to secure the health of people living with HIV. As nonadherence increases risk for drug resistance and viral replication, it is imperative that once people living with HIV begin a particular medication regimen, that regimen remains stable.[32]

Participants also made specific recommendations related to working with those at high risk for HIV infection and those already living with HIV/AIDS. These included expanding activities that target people

---

32. Geletko, S.M., & Poulakos, M.N. (2002). Pharmaceutical services in an HIV clinic. *American Journal of Health-System Pharmacy 50(8)*, 709–13.

living with HIV for primary and secondary prevention, building the skills of HIV positive individuals to disclose their HIV status, and improving negotiation skills for safer sex practices with drug-using partners.

G. Improve and Expand Surveillance Data

"Health data on race and ethnicity must be collected uniformly throughout the United States. To date, one-third of all States throughout our country have yet to break out Asian and Pacific Islanders as a separate category. Until this happens, we will never know the true extent of the epidemic in our communities."

—San Francisco, California community discussion

HIV/AIDS surveillance is critical to HIV prevention efforts: The more we know about populations affected by HIV, the more effective our approach for targeted HIV prevention and improved health outcomes. Recommendations regarding HIV surveillance focused primarily on increasing the specificity in which data are gathered. This includes:

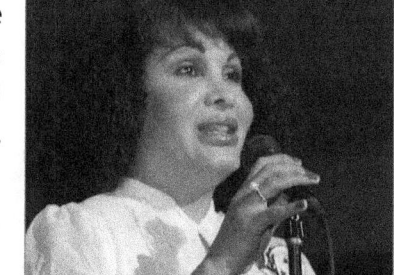

- Increasing demographic categories for race and gender, and
- Collecting a detailed history during testing encounters.

More detailed surveillance categories across local, State, and national data was repeatedly echoed in Web and hard-copy submissions, as well as community discussions. These data are recognized as important tools for creating better strategies for preventing HIV and improving outreach to bring infected persons into care. Many individuals recommended that surveillance data better target specific demographic groups.

Several participants remarked upon improving the accuracy of HIV surveillance information. Statements like, "Include transpeople in collected data on HIV" and "Do not mis-categorize transgender women as MSM," were common across community discussions. We heard from Native Americans and Asian and Pacific Islanders requesting they not be categorized as "other" in surveillance data. Arab Americans asked that they be recognized separately and not classified as "White." African immigrants discussed their unique challenges that set them apart from African-Americans.

H. Summary

We received a variety of specific proposals for reducing HIV incidence. By far, we heard most about the need for a wide-scale and multifaceted HIV prevention campaign to engage the American public.

Targeted efforts for specific populations were also championed during the community discussions, including comprehensive sex education for youth, clean injection equipment for injection drug users, and greater availability of condoms for all groups. It was also a common recommendation that targeted prevention efforts should be accompanied with more accurate surveillance that reflects the diversity of communities.

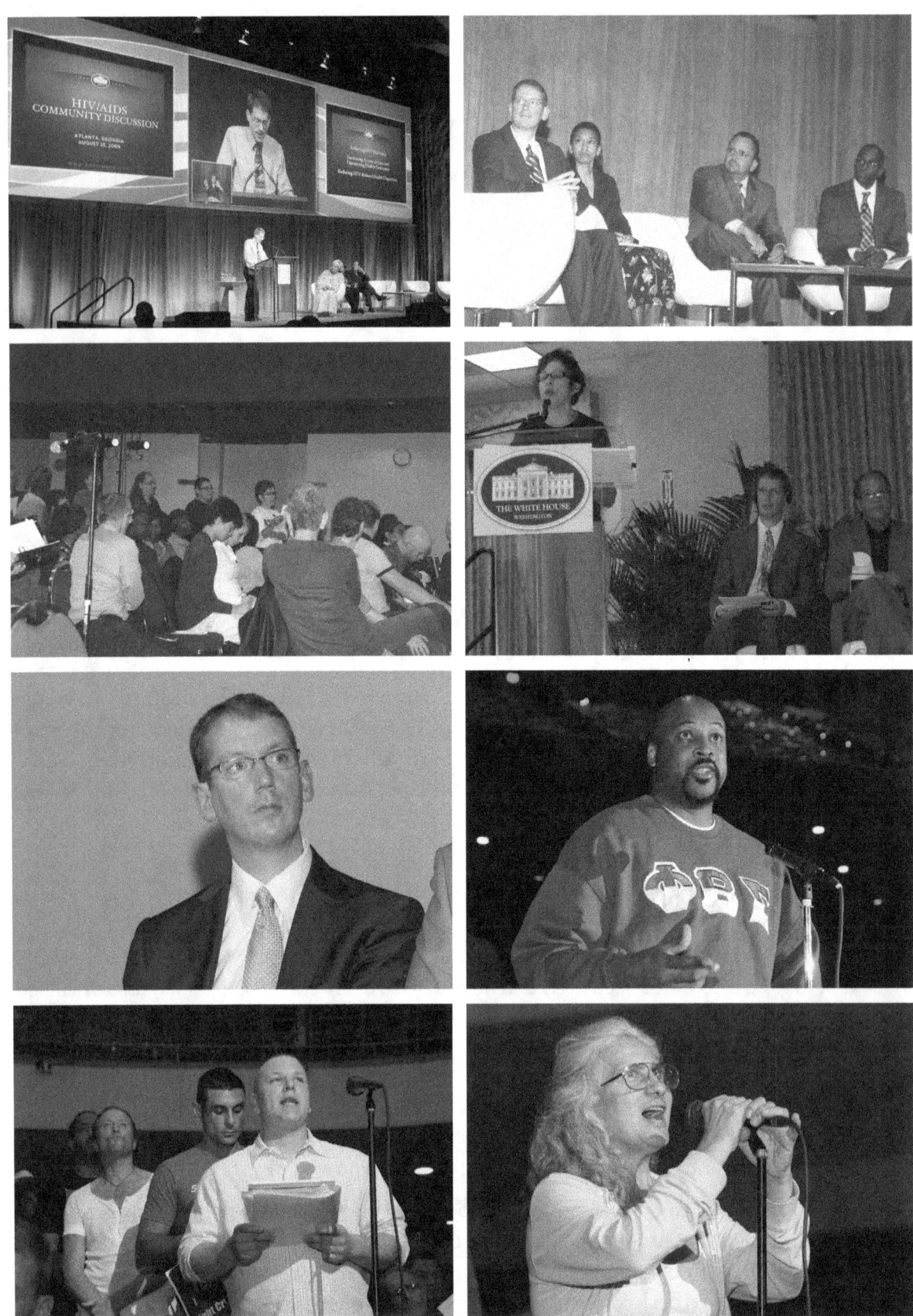

Increasing Access to Care and Optimizing Health Outcomes

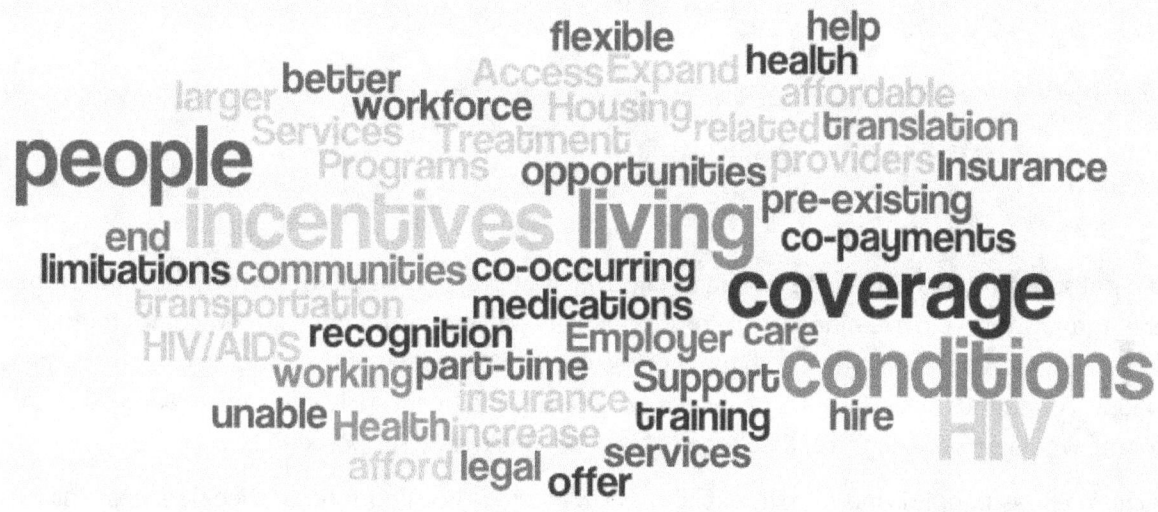

Increasing access to care and improving health outcomes requires coordination in a number of arenas. When people enter care late and have problems staying in care, they suffer poorer health outcomes. There are social, economic, and other factors that affect access to appropriate care. For example, a lack of permanent or stable housing may result in missed appointments and inadequate adherence.[33] Cultural differences and language skills may equate to difficulty navigating the health care system.[34,35] Workforce shortages, particularly in HIV/AIDS and primary care, may mean fewer available providers, longer waiting times for medical appointments, and more obstacles to accessing care.[36,37,38,39]

---

33. National AIDS Housing Coalition. (2008). *Examining the evidence: the impact of housing on HIV prevention and care.* Retrieved from the NAHC Web site:
http://nationalaidshousing.org/PDF/Summary-Key%20Summit%20Findings.pdf., p. 3.

34. Flores, G. (2006, July 20). Language barriers to health care in the United States. *New England Journal of Medicine,* 355(3), 229–231.

35. Center for Outreach Research and Evaluation, Health & Disability Working Group(2006). Making the connection: promoting engagement and retention in HIV medical care among hard-to-reach populations. *Boston University School of Public Health.* Retrieved from the Boston University Web site:
http://www.bu.edu/hdwg/pdf/projects/LessonLearnedFinal.pdf.

36. Carmichael JK, Deckard DT, Feinberg J et al. American Academy of HIV Medicine, HIV Medicine Association. *Averting a crisis in HIV care: a joint statement of the American Academy of HIV Medicine (AAHIVM) and the HIV Medicine Association (HIVMA) on the HIV medical workforce.* June 2009.

37. Dill, M.J., & Salsberg, E.S. (2008, November). The complexities of physician supply and demand: projections through 2025. Association of American Medical Colleges, Center for Workforce Studies. Retrieved from the AAMC Web site: http://services.aamc.org/publications/showfile.cfm?file=version122.pdf&prd_id=244&prv_id=299&pdf_id=122., p. 10.

38. Gilman B, Hargreaves M, Au M, Kim J; Mathematica Policy Research, Inc. (2009, March 6). *Factors Impacting the Retention of Clinical Providers and Other Key Personnel in Ryan White HIV/AIDS Program Care Settings.*

39. HRSA Bureau of Health Professions. (2006, October). *Physician supply and demand: projections to 2020.* Retrieved from the HRSA Web site: ftp://ftp.hrsa.gov/bhpr/workforce/PhysicianForecastingPaperfinal.pdf.

For many people living with HIV, access to the services needed for improving health is hampered by entrenched barriers to services. ONAP received recommendations drawn from individuals' personal experiences and knowledge concerning removing common barriers to care. Recommendations commonly fell in the following categories:

A. Expand Support Services

"I find that my clients are underserved and lack the needed support services and medical care that affects their health and wellbeing."

—Long Beach, California Web submission

It is not surprising that, given the high rates of poverty among people living with HIV, the public urged the Administration to examine the role of support services in optimizing health outcomes for people living with HIV. Considering the combination of poverty and high rates of co-occurring conditions, many people commented that HIV/AIDS treatment extends beyond treating HIV infection, to addressing care for the whole person and the entire range of his or her health and support needs.

Across venues, people living with HIV explained how access to housing, food, and legal services ensured they could focus on managing the disease; how child care and transportation allowed them to keep appointments; how case managers, social workers, and interpreters helped them navigate the health and social services systems; and how support groups and job training meant they could focus not on where they are but on where they wanted to go.

Health Insurance and Access to Treatment

Participants reported that insurance costs remain an extraordinary barrier to prevention and care services for many people living with HIV. A number of individuals stressed the role of cost containment in reducing pressures on public and private insurance programs. Participants also focused on the need to make the Nation's patchwork of public and private programs easier to navigate. They also cited obstacles inherent to enrolling in some programs. "Populations, including homeless U.S. citizens, formerly incarcerated individuals, and legal immigrants have trouble accessing appropriate HIV medical care because they do not possess personal identification documents," noted the Ryan White Medical Providers Coalition in its written recommendations. "Such documents should be made easier to acquire," the group suggested, adding that "jurisdictions that release individuals from incarceration should provide personal identification documents upon release.

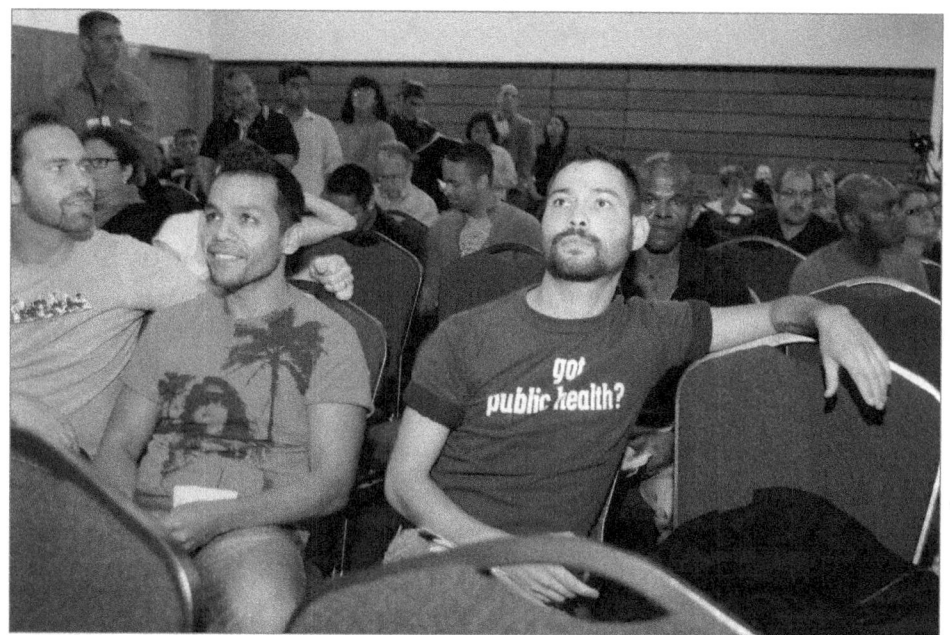

Participants advocated for the removal of coverage limits for particular services such as substance abuse treatment, dental care, and mental health services. In several communities, participants also asked for coverage for hormone therapy treatments that have not been covered historically. Pre-existing conditions and their potential to negatively impact health coverage and health outcomes was also echoed across community discussions. As the Staten Island Ryan White Part B HIV CARE Network wrote, "[We] support language in health insurance reform legislation prohibiting companies from refusing coverage for an individual based on their medical history or health risk."

One of the most frequently repeated policy recommendations was to address the Medicare Part D coverage gap, often referred to as the Medicare "donut hole." Once Part D enrollees surpass the prescription drug coverage limit, they are responsible for 100 percent of the total drug costs until they reach the "catastrophic coverage threshold."[40] As a Florida HIV pharmacist described, "Many Medicare D clients self ration their drugs because of the donut hole. They split tablets. They skip days. They skip drugs. This can lead to viral resistance. It can lead to secondary infections. It can lead to infecting others with the resistant virus all of which could cause or increase health costs later on."

Some community discussion attendees called for a more rapid FDA approval process for HIV treatments. Other health care advocates asked for additional policies to improve access to the Ryan White AIDS Drug Assistance Program (ADAP) and Medicare Part D.

Participants also asked for less stringent eligibility requirements and for shorter waiting periods for some programs. "Patients…must wait 24 months after qualifying for SSDI [Social Security Income Disability Insurance] for their Medicare coverage to come into force. The waiting period creates gaps in care for these patients and Ryan White funds are not always readily available to fill these gaps. Such waiting periods should be abolished so that individuals have seamless access to care."

---

40. Hoadley, J., & Hargrave, E. (2009, November). Medicare Part D 2010 data spotlight: the coverage gap. KFF. Retrieved from the KFF Web site: http://www.kff.org/medicare/upload/8008.pdf., p. 1.

Housing

"[W]hen we talk about housing first, it really is housing first. If you do not have a place to live it is really difficult to even think about medication, to think about medical appointments, to think about behavior changes."

—San Francisco, California community discussion

According to the National AIDS Housing Coalition, an estimated 50 percent of persons infected with HIV will need some sort of housing assistance over the course of their illness.[41] Lack of stable housing can pose enormous barriers to staying in care and treatment adherence. Thus, housing is often viewed as a health care issue. "Acquiring and maintaining stable housing has long been recognized as an important component in the response to HIV/AIDS," noted one New York State resident. "The lack of a home undermines sound nutrition and HIV treatment adherence, makes contact with health care providers difficult, and makes employment problematic."

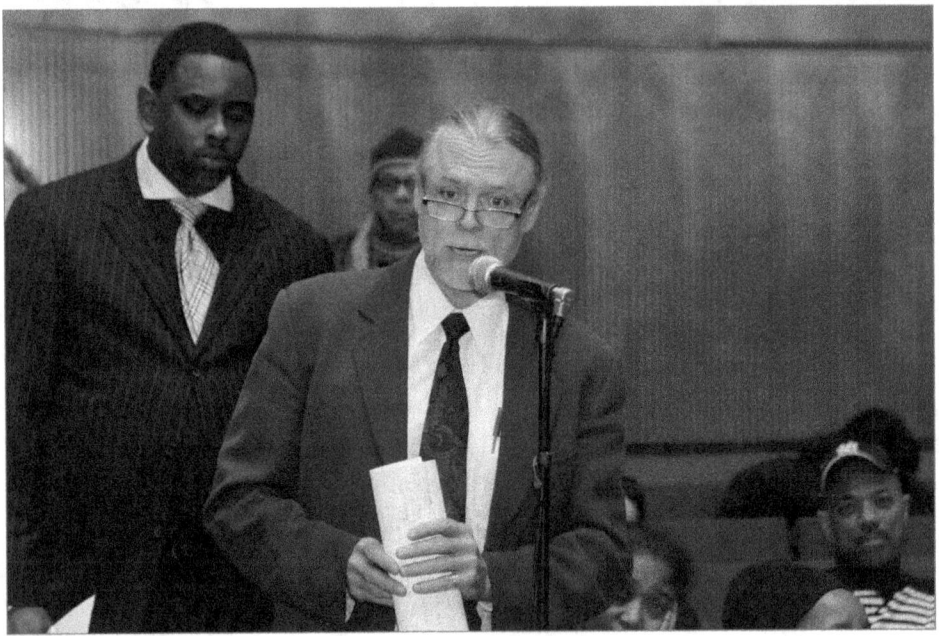

Many persons who are homeless, in transitional housing, in shelters, and assisted living came out to the community discussions. In urban areas, they voiced their concerns about the high cost of living. In San Francisco, for example, people discussed the challenges of living in the country's second-highest-priced housing market and making ends meet with current levels of Federal income support. Others discussed the need for longer grace periods before eviction for persons who are sick or recently disabled. "One thing that we can do is have a national standard of 120 days notice to evict a senior, disabled, or catastrophically ill tenant," said one speaker.

---

41. National AIDS Housing Coalition. (2008). *HOPWA 2009 need*. Retrieved from the NAHC Web site: http://nationalaidshousing.org/PDF/FY09HOPWANeedPaper.pdf., p. 1.

Around the Nation, many members of the public have called for greater funding for housing assistance. In addition, many called for a more streamlined application process for the Housing Opportunities for Persons with AIDS (HOPWA) program. The public also requested that housing policy reflects the unique needs of populations such as at-risk youth or youth living with HIV, persons recently released from correctional settings, and transgender individuals.

Job Training/Employment Services

> "Resources should be committed to enhance economic stability through education, jobs, and leadership training."
>
> —Washington, D.C. Web submission

HIV affects the most vulnerable in our society. Nearly 60 percent of individuals receiving care from the Ryan White HIV/AIDS Program had household incomes at or below the Federal poverty level.[42] Moreover, studies have shown that among individuals living with HIV, educational attainment has a direct correlation with health outcomes.[43]

Participants at various community discussions advised the Administration that these results underscored the need for increased access to job training and employment services. Participants made specific suggestions to capitalize on the unique experiences many have acquired through their work as peer counselors. They also noted that while many would like to work, HIV compromises their ability to do so on a regular basis.

Others explained the employment dilemma faced by persons currently receiving disability benefits who fear entering the workforce and losing needed disability benefits. "I want to continue to contribute as much as possible by working," explained a Seattle, Washington man. "But work is largely an either/or situation. I am considering returning to disability."

Participants also voiced worries about being unable to afford private health insurance or being denied health insurance due to a pre-existing condition. They called for:

- An end to insurance coverage limitations related to pre-existing conditions,
- More affordable health care coverage,
- Programs and incentives to help people living with HIV who are working, but unable to afford co-payments and medications, and
- Employer incentives to hire people living with HIV and to offer flexible, part-time opportunities.

---

42. HRSA. (2008). *The power of connections*. Retrieved from the HRSA Web site: http://hab.hrsa.gov/publications/progressreport08/2008ProgressReport.pdf., p. 39.

43. Marc, L.G., Testa, M.A., Walker, A.M., Robbins, G.K., Shafer, R.W., Anderson, N.B., & Berkman, L.F. (2007, August). Educational attainment and response to HAART during initial therapy for HIV-1 infection. *Journal of Psychosomatic Research, 63(2)*, 207–216.

Comments highlighted that employment and job training services are especially important for people transitioning from corrections institutions. Research indicates that each year, about one in four people living with HIV spend time in a correctional facility,[44] and participants at the community discussions frequently referenced the unique employment challenges of ex-offenders. Participants discussed the importance of re-entry programs that help ex-offenders succeed and that keep them from returning to the environment and circumstances that resulted in their initial incarceration.

One New York State man explained his recommendation through his life experience in a study group:

> "[The doctor] studied two approaches to re-entry of formerly incarcerated [people living with HIV]. One group received minimal transition planning. They relied on welfare and safe houses once released. The other was provided with comprehensive transitional support, including access to education, job training, and transitional housing. Ten years later all the members of the first group are dead. The second group, we are still here. I was part of that second group. I am now a successful community advocate and a retired health educator for the State. I am proof of the success of a holistic approach to HIV."

Some respondents called for job training to begin while individuals are still incarcerated. Others recommended training as part of a re-entry program. Many participants pleaded for government incentives for businesses to hire ex-offenders and for apprenticeships to train this population for long-term employment.

Transportation

> "People in rural areas may face tremendous barriers to health care. Two of those barriers are stigma and transportation. Transportation would not be as big an issue if we had more doctors trained to treat HIV."
>
> —Finger Lakes Region, New York recommendation

Transportation issues in many rural and suburban areas involve lack of infrastructure, and people living with HIV in urban areas face unique challenges related to transportation as well. Since people living with HIV are disproportionately poor, even accessible public transportation systems may be too expensive for indigent individuals and families.

---

44. Okie, S. (2007, January 11). Sex, drugs, prisons, and HIV. *New England Journal of Medicine*, 356(2),106.

The need for transportation support has long been a factor affecting access to care. Transportation services for accessing medical care are funded through Medicaid and can be funded through the Ryan White Program. Since Ryan White prioritizes funding core medical services, however, rising prevalence in many communities has forced cuts in funding for transportation and other nonmedical support services.

Many individuals have called for increasing funding for transportation services for people living with HIV. Still others have recommended improving the country's transportation infrastructure and public transit systems, especially in more rural and suburban communities. These areas have fewer providers, often requiring patients to travel long distances for care. As a Columbia, South Carolina resident explained, "There is just not enough means of getting from point A to point B."

Legal Services

"Many experts now recognize that law and legal counseling can play a pivotal role in stemming the spread of HIV by ensuring access to public and private resources essential to preventing and managing HIV effectively."

—Washington, D.C. Web submission

From rural residents to those living in the country's most populated cities, advocates explained the critical role legal services play in helping clients gain access to and stay in care, remain in their homes, and counter discriminatory employment practices and other issues people living with HIV face.

One New York City-based organization stated, "Since the creation of the Ryan White CARE Act,[45] thousands of [people living with HIV] have accessed legal services that have enabled them to obtain medically appropriate housing, access to medical benefits and services, fight discrimination, and make appropriate end-of-life care decisions." Several individuals spoke critically of current Ryan White policies that limit the scope of legal services that can be funded through the Ryan White HIV/AIDS Program. Some individuals called for States to expand the legal services they cover through Ryan White, whereas others advocated for clearer guidance from HRSA that explicitly defines a broad range of legal services that can be covered.

"The unnecessarily narrow definition of the scope of legal services is depriving PLWHAs [people living with HIV/AIDS] of crucial support services, including such fundamental assistance as eviction prevention," asserted South Brooklyn Legal Services. One individual added, "We have the capacity to represent people in asylum cases who have been forced to leave their own country for being tortured because of HIV and because of their…sexual relationships … [but under the current Ryan White definition] we are not allowed to do so."

---

45. The Ryan White Comprehensive AIDS Resources Emergency (CARE) Act is now referred to as the Ryan White HIV/AIDS Program.

Translation Services

"There must be a plan [that] ensures translation is always accessible and available to all people with HIV/AIDS."

—Philadelphia, Pennsylvania Web submission

> **Language Line**
>
> While many urban areas have access to an array of interpreters and some larger medical facilities have them or bilingual staff on hand, smaller or more traditional settings cannot afford this luxury. Many are, therefore, turning to Language Line, an organization offering live, confidential medical interpretation services by telephone in over 170 languages.
>
> (To learn more, visit http://www.languageline.com/page/industry_healthcare/ or call 1-800-752-6096.)

Access to language services and translated documents can help facilitate effective communication between people living with HIV and their providers. The capacity to communicate with clients in the language in which they are most comfortable is an important component of cultural competency. Individuals identified language and translation services as critical needs associated with optimizing health outcomes.

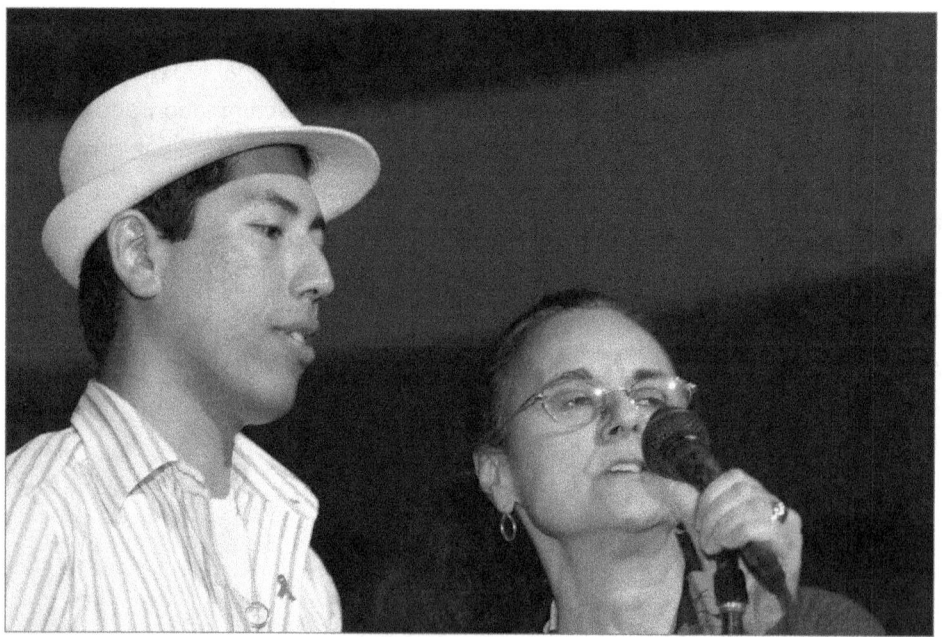

A Rochester, New York man stated, "I am an Asian gay man who is deaf. I am speaking to you through an interpreter. When I was diagnosed, I went to the doctor's office. The sign language interpreter didn't know the medical words used for HIV. Besides being emotionally distraught over being HIV positive, a non-English speaking person faces confusion and frustration from not being able to communicate with the people who are trying to help."

As a project manager at the Asian and Pacific Islander Coalition explained, "New York [City] is a city of immigrants. Asian and Pacific Islanders make up 12 percent of the population. Seventy-two percent of this population group is foreign born and…49 percent speak English less than very well…[and need] access to culturally and linguistically competent services."

According to a *New England Journal of Medicine* study, 22.3 million Americans have limited English proficiency—a number that has grown in recent years.[46] According to one study, nearly one-half (46 percent) of emergency room cases of patients with limited English proficiency had no interpreter assistance.[47] This lack of available interpreters is directly related to workforce shortages, lack of clinician training with interpreters, and lack of reimbursement for interpreter services. Yet access to these services has shown to have a positive improvement in patient satisfaction and overall health outcomes.[48,49]

Case Management

"AIDS case management services allow people to access primary health care and to maintain their dignity and respect."

—Los Angeles, California community discussion

Case managers are an important resource for linking people to services, coordinating care, and ensuring retention in care. Case managers are often the persons with whom people living with HIV have the most direct contact. They are involved in making referrals, tracking follow-up, and monitoring patient utilization and outcomes, and they can play a significant role in determining if patients stay in care. Case managers often work closely with HIV/AIDS and primary care providers as part of a comprehensive team approach.[50]

---

46. Flores, G. (2006, July 20). Language barriers to health care in the United States. *New England Journal of Medicine,* 355(3), 229.

47. Baker DW, Parker RM, Williams MV, Coates WC, Pitkin K. (1996). Use and effectiveness of interpreters in an emergency department. *Journal of the American Medical Association*.275(10), 783–8.

48. Flores, G. (2006, July 20). Language barriers to health care in the United States. *New England Journal of Medicine,* 355(3), 231.

49. Flores, G., Laws, M.B., Mayo, S.J., Zuckerman, B., Abreu, M., Medina, L., & Hardt, E.J. (2003, January). Errors in medical interpretation and their potential clinical consequences in pediatric encounters. *Pediatrics,* 111(1), 13.

50. CDC. (2006). *Demonstration projects for health departments and community-based organizations (CBOs): antiretroviral treatment access study (ARTAS) II: linkage to HIV care.* Retrieved from the CDC Web site: http://www.cdc.gov/hiv/topics/prev_prog/ahp/resources/factsheets/pdf/ARTASII.pdf., p. 1.

As a Long Island, New York man explained,

"HIV/AIDS medical care often involves a complex continuum of care. Even those of us who have been living with the disease for decades require the assistance of a case manager to help navigate the system. In addition, as we live longer, new issues emerge that we need guidance on. We cannot stress enough the importance of our case managers, of having someone who knows us, knows our needs, and knows the continuum of care. We urge the Federal government to continue the support of community-based case management programs for all people living with HIV, not just the newly diagnosed. We also recognize that there is very high turnover rates among case managers and encourage the Federal government to support programs to increase retention and continuing education for our case managers."

Case managers can also link patients to population-specific services, such as assisting HIV-positive mothers in identifying and gaining access to child-care services, or helping to enroll clients in programs like WIC (the Special Supplemental Nutrition Program for Women, Infants, and Children). Many participants at the community discussions called for increased access to supportive services like these as a step toward both decreasing no-show rates for medical appointments and increasing patient adherence to treatment. Availability of child care services for mothers may help improve patient retention,[51] while access to nutritional services can play an important role in improving medication absorption and malnutrition.[52]

Case managers may be able to help assess patient needs and work to ensure patient access of necessary services. These services may range from oral health care to housing assistance and anything in between.[53] Whether they are medical or nonmedical case managers, these individuals play an important role in assisting people living with HIV. As a Fort Lauderdale community discussion participant summarized, "Without the support that I have gotten from my case manager...I probably would not be here today."

---

51. CORE/HDWG. (2006). Making the connection: promoting engagement and retention in HIV medical care among hard-to-reach populations. , *Boston University School of Public Health*. Retrieved from the Boston University Web site: http://www.bu.edu/hdwg/pdf/projects/LessonLearnedFinal.pdf.

52. American Dietetic Association. (2004). Position of the American Dietetic Association and the Dietitians of Canada: Nutrition intervention in the care of persons with human immunodeficiency virus infection. *Journal of the American Dietetic Association*, 104, 1427.

53. HRSA. (2008, November). *Care Action. Retrieved from the HRSA Web site*: http://hab.hrsa.gov/publications/november2008/November08.pdf., p. 3.

B. Include Chronic Disease Management in Overall Health Care Delivery

"Our nationally recognized medication management program has resulted in…the prevention of chronic disease progression."

—Smyrna, Georgia Web submission

Many participants at the community discussions urged the Government to seize the opportunity presented by health care reform legislation to cover all Americans and create a framework for chronic disease management. "All too often, people suffering from multiple chronic conditions receive little to no coordination of their health care from the various specialists that they regularly interact with. Adapt chronic health care models that emphasize outpatient primary care, patient education, and multiple-condition health care coordination," urged a Harlem, New York organization.

High Rates of Co-occurring Conditions Among People Living with HIV Requires Improved Access to Care

The rates of some health conditions among people living with HIV are related to the long-term effects of HIV and its treatment such as lipoatrophy and lipodystrophy. But high rates of poverty and stigma and poor access to regular medical care also contribute to HIV-related disparities as well.

The prevalence of hepatitis C among people living with HIV may be as high as 30 percent and as high as 90 percent among people infected with HIV through injection drug use.

Studies on post-traumatic stress disorder in people living with HIV have found prevalence rates from between 30 and 50 percent; approximately 60 percent of individuals meeting diagnostic criteria were untreated for their condition.

People living with HIV have high rates of oral health problems, a contributor to poor nutrition and the capacity to adhere to treatment regimens, and they are at disproportionate risk for medical concerns associated with the aging process.

Sources: Gennaro, S., Naidoo, S., & Berthold, P. (2008). Oral health and HIV/AIDS. *American Journal of Maternal/Child Nursing, 33(1)*, 50-7.
Israelski, D.M., Prentiss, D.E., Lubega, S., Balmas, G., Garcia, P., Muhammad, M.,… Koopman, C. (2007). Psychiatric co-morbidity in vulnerable populations receiving primary care for HIV/AIDS. *AIDS Care*, 19(2), 220-5.
School of Dentistry, Louisiana State University Health Sciences Center. (2007). *HIV+ outpatient overview*.
Sherman, K.E., Rouster, S.D., Chung, R.T., & Rajicic, N. (2002). Hepatitis C virus prevalence among patients infected with human immunodeficiency virus: a cross-sectional analysis of the US adult AIDS Clinical Trials Group. *Clinical Infectious Diseases 34(6)*, 831-837.
Sulkowski, M.S., & Thomas, (2003). D.L.. Hepatitis C in the HIV-infected person. *Annals of Internal Medicine 138(3)*, 197-207.
Thomas, D.L.(2002). Hepatitis C and human immunodeficiency virus infection. *Hepatology 36 (5 suppl 1)*, S201-9.

Chronic disease management is a comprehensive, coordinated approach for addressing the health care needs of the patient. Such an approach is intended to improve health, lower incidence of comorbidities and medical complications, slow disease progression, and potentially reduce health disparities among people living with HIV. "Part C [of the Ryan White HIV/AIDS Program] clearly needs more funding to provide direct medical care in the chronic disease model," mentioned an Albuquerque, New Mexico medical director.

In addition to expressing support for chronic disease management coverage in general, many recommendations focused on specific services that such an approach could encompass. In particular, the importance of preventive health care was repeatedly highlighted. Participants at the community discussions promoted the use of peer counselors, noting the proven value of this approach in educating patients about living with HIV disease and its comorbidities, as well as supporting treatment adherence. "We need more prevention-with-positives interventions," said one participant. "Utilize peer-based models to retain women living with HIV in care," added another.

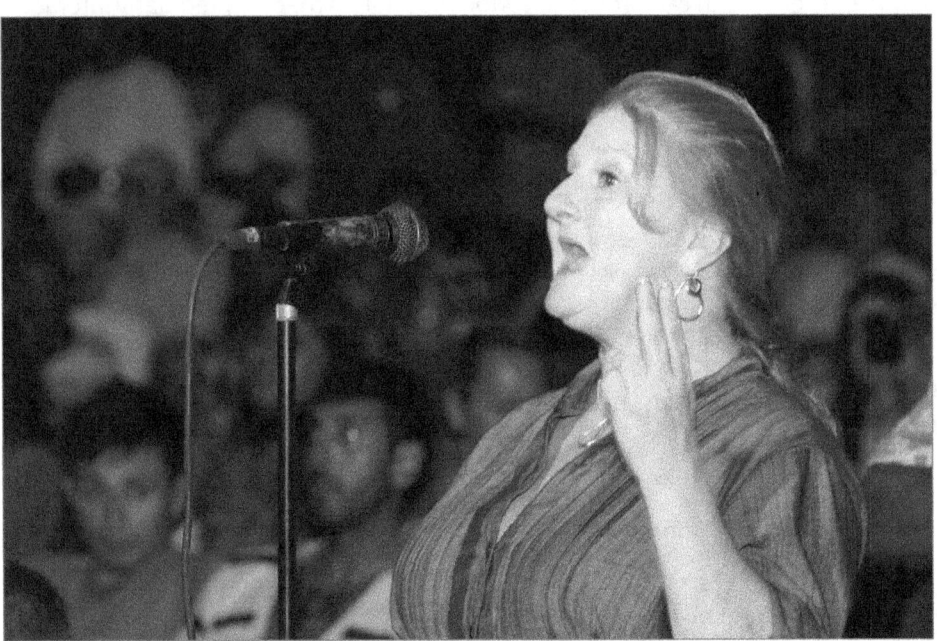

At the Puerto Rico community discussion as well as many others, individuals discussed how improved treatment has helped HIV evolve into a chronic disease. As the Services & Advocacy for Gay, Lesbian, bisexual & Transgender Elders organization explained, "If current trends in infection rates remain stable, in less than 10 years, one-half of all people living with HIV in the United States will be over age 50." The AIDS Community Research Initiative of America (ACRIA) added that, "As people with HIV grow older, they become prey to the same ailments faced by their HIV-negative brothers and sisters, such as arthritis, cardiovascular disease, diabetes, and dementia." As the HIV population ages—whether as long-term survivors or from contracting the disease later in life—participants called for increased care coordination with conditions that commonly occur with aging.

Comments frequently included the need for increasing access to a multidisciplinary team of specialists to ensure providers can address the unique needs of not only the older population but of all persons managing HIV.

C. Recognize and Treat Co-occurring Conditions

"Many Americans who are at risk of contracting HIV are also at risk of contracting viral hepatitis…Viral hepatitis is the most common cause of liver cancer, which is one of the most lethal, expensive, and fastest rising cancers in the United States."

—Hepatitis C Appropriations Partnership Web submission

HIV/AIDS services providers are working in a world with growing medical need. While treatment of HIV/AIDS with antiretroviral therapy has been a success, the incidence of comorbidities associated with aging and long-term survival has increased. Moreover, people living with HIV may be at heightened risk for other conditions, including addiction, mental illness, tuberculosis, and hepatitis C, as well as certain metabolic and other disorders such as heart disease. These conditions fuel a high level of demand for services.

In the HIV Costs and Services Utilization Study (HCSUS), one-half of adults with HIV had symptoms of a psychiatric disorder; 19 percent had signs of substance abuse, and 13 percent had co-occurring substance abuse and mental illness.[54] Yet approximately one-half of people living with HIV who have depression have undiagnosed and untreated conditions.[55] The implications of untreated mental illness are severe. Psychiatric disorders can pose barriers to medical care and negatively affect medication adherence. Several studies have found that depression, trauma, stress, and anxiety can lead to increased disease progression and mortality.[56,57,58,59]

Recent research on people living with HIV being treated for depression found that use of selective serotonin reuptake inhibitors (SSRIs) not only improved mental health but had a direct correlation on improved antiretroviral adherence and decreased viral load.[60] These findings echo the calls of many respondents for increased screening for—and access to—mental health services for people living with HIV, which they stated is highly disproportionate among this population. "Treatment of mental illnesses has to be one of the top priorities in the fight against HIV/AIDS," said a Web respondent from San Juan, Puerto Rico. "[There is] a dire need for psychiatric, substance abuse, and other mental health services

---

54. Bing, E.G., Burnman, M.A., Longshore, D., Fleishman, J.A., Sherbourne, C.D., London, A.S,& Shapiro, M. (2001, August). Psychiatric disorders and drug use among human immunodeficiency virus-infected adults in the United States. *Archives of General Psychiatry*, 58(8), 721–728.

55. Lesser, J. (2008). Role of depression, stress, and trauma in HIV disease progression. *Psychosomatic Medicine*, 70, 539-545.

56. Treisman, G.J., Angelina, A.F., & Hutton, H.E. (2001). Psychiatric issues in the management of patients with HIV infection. *Journal of the American Medical Society*, 286, 2857–2864.

57. Lesser, J. (2008). Role of depression, stress, and trauma in HIV disease progression. Psychosomatic Medicine, 70, 539.

58. Starace, F., Ammassari, A., Trotta, M.P., Murri, R., DeLongis, P., Izzo, C,& Antinori, A. (2002). Depression is a risk factor for suboptimal adherence to highly active antiretroviral therapy. *Journal of Acquired Immune Deficiency Syndromes*, 31(S136-S139), S136.

59. Whetten, K., Reif, S., Whetten, R., Murphy-McMillian, L.K. (2008). Trama, mental health, distrust, and stigma among HIV-positive persons: implications for effective care. *Psychosomatic Medicine*, 70, 531.

60. Horberg, M.A., Silverberg, M.J, Hurley, L.B.,Towner, W.J., Kelin, D.B., Bersoff-Matcha, S.,& Kovach, D.A. (2008, March 1). Effects of depression and selective serotonin reuptake inhibitor use on adherence to highly active antiretroviral therapy and on clinical outcomes in HIV-infected patients. *Journal of Acquired Immune Deficiency Syndromes*, 47(3), 384–90.

in the community," wrote a doctor from Chicago, Illinois. "There are no resources for mental health or counseling with respect to HIV/AIDS. I asked my doctor after I was diagnosed over a year-and-a-half ago for a referral to some sort of counseling. He had none to offer," explained a Mississippi man. We need more mental health and substance abuse treatment and funding for those treatments," added a Fort Lauderdale, Florida physician.

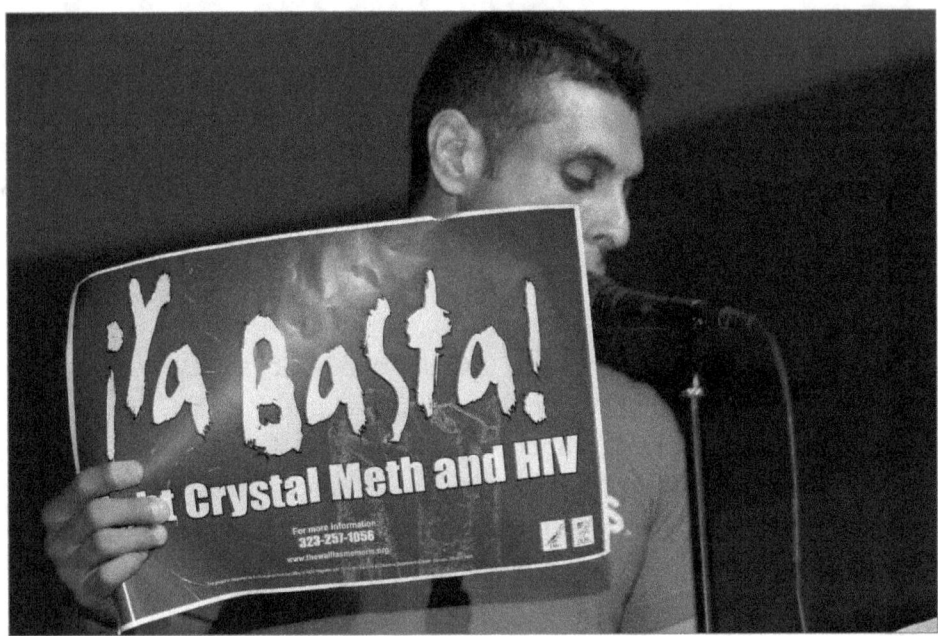

Some drugs, such as methamphetamine, can a cause cognitive impairment,[61] lead to depression (due to damage of dopamine receptors),[62] increase HIV viral replication,[63] and remove protective mucosa making people susceptible to a variety of pathogens including HIV.[64,65] Other drug-taking activities, like injection drug use, have long been recognized for its role in HIV transmission.[66] Injection drug use has also been shown to fuel health conditions like hepatitis C. Hepatitis C may interfere with HIV treatment and may lead to increased progression of liver disease.[67] End stage liver disease is now a major cause of

---

61. Rippeth, J.D., Heaton, R.K., Carey, C.L, Marcotte, T.D., Moore, D.J., Gonzalez, R., & Grant, I. (2004). Methamphetamine dependence increases risk of neuropsychological impairment in HIV infected persons. *Journal of the International Neuropsychological Society, 10(1)*, 1–14.

62. National Institute of Drug Abuse. (2006, September). *Methamphetamine abuse and addiction.* Retrieved from the NIDA Web site: www.nida.nih.gov/PDF/RRMetham.pdf., p. 5.

63. Gavrilin, M.A., Mathes, L.E., Podell, M. (2002). Methamphetamine enhances cell-associated feline immunodeficiency virus replication in astrocytes. *Journal for Neurovirology, 8(3)*, 240–249.

64. CDC (2007, January). *Methamphetamine use and risk for HIV/AIDS.* Retrieved from the CDC Web site: http://www.cdc.gov/hiv/resources/factsheets/meth.htm.

65. Yeon, P., & Albrecht, H. (2008, February). Crystal methamphetamine and HIV/AIDS. *AIDS Clinical Care, 20(2)*, 2–4.

66. National Institute of Drug Abuse. (2006, March). *Research report series: HIV/AIDS.* Retrieved from the NIDA Web site: http://www.drugabuse.gov/PDF/RRhiv.pdf., p. 3.

67. CDC. (2005, November). *Coinfection with HIV and hepatitis C virus.* Retrieved from the CDC Web site: http://www.cdc.gov/hiv/resources/Factsheets/coinfection.htm.

death among persons infected with HIV.[68,69,70] Infection with HIV is also the strongest known risk factor for progression from latent tuberculosis to active (or contagious) tuberculosis.[71,72]

As a Providence, Rhode Island respondent wrote, "Prisoners face an enormous burden of co-occurring disorders such as mental illness, addiction, viral hepatitis, and sexually transmitted diseases. Another person said, "Correctional settings represent a major opportunity…[for] prison and jail-based screening, treatment, and linkage to care." This comment came from one of the many participants who stressed the need to better utilize key points of entry[73] to identify, address, and treat co-infections. In many recommendations, respondents emphasized the risk of infection with multiple sexually transmitted diseases. Sexually transmitted diseases such as syphilis infection are shown to increase HIV viral load and heighted transmissibility of HIV.[74] People living with HIV may also experience more severe reactions to particular sexually transmitted infections, such as gonorrhea and herpes, due to their weakened immune systems.[75]

D. Increase the Number of HIV Care Providers and HIV/AIDS Education and Training

"As an internist who just completed residency, I feel very comfortable treating the complications of HIV in a hospital setting but have limited knowledge in treating outpatient HIV. In my residency program, patients who were diagnosed with HIV were transferred to the Infectious Disease clinics. As a new physician I am excited and honored to work with this population, but I do feel overwhelmed at times by all of the information I need to learn."

—Virgin Islands Web submission

---

68. Sherman, K.E., Rouster, S.D., Chung, R.T., & Rajicic, N. (2002). Hepatitis C virus prevalence among patients infection with human immunodeficiency virus: a cross-sectional analysis of the US adult AIDS Clinical Trial Group. *Clinical Infectious Diseases, 34,* 831.

69. Sulkowski, M.S., & Thomas, D.L. (2003). Hepatitis C in the HIV-infected person. *Annals of Internal Medicine, 138(3),* 197.

70. Thomas Thomas, D.L. (2002). Hepatitis C and human immunodeficiency virus infection. *Hepatology, 36(supplement 5),* S201–9.

71. CDC. (2009, June 1). *Tuberculosis (TB): general information.* Retrieved from the CDC Web site: http://www.cdc.gov/tb/publications/factsheets/general/tb.pdf., p. 2.

72. CDC. (2009, June 1). *Tuberculosis (TB): TB and HIV coinfection.* Retrieved from the CDC Web site: http://www.cdc.gov/tb/topic/TBHIVcoinfection/default.htm.

73. Key points of entry include emergency rooms, substance abuse treatment programs, detoxification centers, adult and juvenile detention facilities, sexually transmitted disease clinics, HIV counseling and testing sites, mental health programs and homeless shelters.

74. Buchacz, K., Patel, P., & Taylor, M. (2004). Syphilis increases HIV viral load and decreases CD4 cell counts in HIV-infected patients with new syphilis infections. *AIDS, 18(15),* 2075–2079.

75. Sowadsky R. (2009, March). The HIV-STD connection. *The Body.* Retrieved from the Body Web site: http://www.thebody.com/content/prev/art2283.html.

This doctor's experience reinforces findings from a 2004 HIV Medicine Association survey. The survey included 729 first-year internal medicine residents in the 10 States with the highest HIV prevalence. One-half (51 percent) of respondents said their residency had not prepared them for HIV medicine.[76] The need to increase the breadth of HIV training was an issue raised across community discussions. Participants stressed the importance of improving capacity, increasing the number of providers, and creating a workforce where HIV education extends to all health professions.

Increase Capacity in Minority Communities

"Community-based organizations are in the position to directly address issues prevalent [in] their own communities," said one respondent from Stockton, California. Access to technical assistance and training can ensure that community-based organizations (CBOs) have increased capacity to address local challenges and barriers to care.

Organizations based within the communities they seek to serve may be uniquely positioned to garner community buy-in and local leadership support. This factor is of particular importance to communities that have been disenfranchised and suffered discrimination, such as racial and ethnic minorities. "Let people of color develop their own messages that work, not outside people telling them how and what they need to do. Help develop and educate grassroots CBOs and ASOs about how to serve the community they are in," emphasized a Stratford, Connecticut resident.

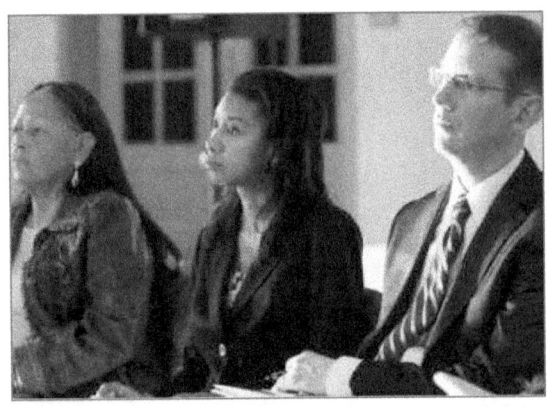

"Accessing and building the capacity of faith-based organizations is also necessary," advised a Cleveland, Ohio minister. The emphasis on training faith-based leaders and engaging faith-based organizations in the fight against HIV/AIDS was stressed as a critical step in reaching minorities, particularly Black and Latino communities.

Many minority communities in both urban and rural areas have few health care providers due to challenges in recruiting and retaining health care professionals. According to a 2008 survey of Ryan White HIV/AIDS-funded clinics, lack of reimbursement and lack of providers were cited as leading causes preventing recruitment.[77] Although it is unknown what proportion of these surveyed clinics are based in communities of color, Ryan White HIV/AIDS Program clients are overwhelmingly from these communities: 72 percent of clients are racial or ethnic minorities and 89 percent are either uninsured or on a public insurance plan.[78]

---

76. Lubinski C. What We Know About the Workforce in HIV/AIDS. Presentation at the HIV/AIDS Workforce Meeting of HRSA, HIV/AIDS Bureau, Rockville, MD, September 15–16, 2008.

77. Infectious Diseases Society of America. (2009). Report: Federal HIV policies need to keep pace with scientific advancements. *ISDA News.19(4)*. Available at: http://news.idsociety.org/idsa/issues/2009-04-01/12.html.

78. HRSA. (2008). *The power of connections*. Retrieved from the HRSA Web site: http://hab.hrsa.gov/publications/progressreport08/2008ProgressReport.pdf., p. 38.

In minority neighborhoods, community organizations often serve as the pathway into the health care system. It is no surprise, then, that many participants at the community discussions called for increased HIV/AIDS training for organizations providing social services.

"Build capacity for community-based organizations that work primarily with women and support providers that have demonstrated core competence in working with [this population]," requested one San Francisco Web respondent. "As part of the consultation and community engagement, ONAP should ensure that tribes and Native American CBOs receive technical and capacity building assistance," suggested another participant.

Build a Bigger, Better Workforce

"…Patients need HIV medication. They also need access to the health care providers that can prescribe the medication."

—Birmingham, Alabama Web submission

"More than a third of U.S. physicians in practice are age 55 or older and likely to retire in the next 10 to 15 years. The aging of the physician workforce will be a key factor limiting future growth of the health care system."[79] Several comments discussed how the shortage of providers working in HIV/AIDS and primary care stands to pose significant barriers to people living with HIV and the health infrastructure in place to care for these persons. A hospital worker in St. Thomas explained that after 30 years of hospital work, there had been no training opportunities in which she could enroll to learn about HIV specialty care. Other participants noted that increasing demands for expanding the scope of HIV/AIDS services, as well as low provider reimbursement rates, is further exacerbating this problem. While these trends exist in many States, participants reminded us that rural communities in the South, in particular, are experiencing acute provider shortages as HIV/AIDS incidence and prevalence increase in this region. A submission from Arkansas summed up many of these comments: "There is a shortage of doctors and medical professionals experienced with treating HIV and it is nearly impossible for many individuals to travel the often long distances to reach those that do exist for adequate treatment and lab work."

Participants across the 14 community discussions were very vocal about the steps the Administration could take to try to curtail the workforce shortage of providers working in HIV/AIDS or primary care. By far, the most recommendations related to government incentives for health professionals (e.g., doctors, nurses, dentists, pharmacists) to enter HIV/AIDS or primary care or to work with HIV-positive persons. Specifically, participants suggested loan repayment or loan forgiveness programs for persons entering into these fields and for those willing to work in high-need communities, including rural towns. "Nobody is going into primary care anymore or HIV, partly because of the costs [and] partly because when they graduate from medical school they owe thousands [or] hundreds of thousands of dollars," said an Albuquerque, New Mexico doctor in favor of loan forgiveness.

---

79. HRSA. HRSA moves to head off health care workforce shortages. (2009, January). *Inside HRSA*. Retrieved from the HRSA Web site: http://newsroom.hrsa.gov/insidehrsa/jan2009/. Accessed November 2009.

As an HIV/AIDS doctor explained,

"Not a lot of docs and health care providers are coming into the business. It does not actually pay terribly well for one thing…so [we need] some kind of program to support the training of physicians and other health care workers in the area of HIV medicine."

The American Academy of HIV Medicine suggested, "The Administration should provide for expanded opportunities for medical, PA [physician assistant], and NP [nurse practitioner] students to seek practice opportunities in HIV medicine as part of their training and to pursue clinical fellowships after their residency…to draw some students into HIV care that would not otherwise focus on the field." The American Association of Colleges of Nursing echoed this recommendation and highlighted the dwindling number of nurses in HIV/AIDS care because of the unavailability of training.

Curricula and Improved Education of Providers

Quality of life and life expectancy for people living with HIV have improved dramatically since the advent of highly active antiretroviral therapy. Yet treating the disease remains complex. Today, providers across a number of health disciplines are now caring for and treating people living with HIV. This factor has resulted in a call to teach all health professionals, regardless of medical specialty, about HIV/AIDS. Some participants focused on the need to provide HIV/AIDS education to individuals working in fields ranging from education, law, social work, psychology, and others.

> **Keeping Providers Abreast of Latest Research Findings**
>
> The debate on the optimal time to begin treatment has been ongoing for some times. A number of Web submissions highlighted recent research on earlier initiation of antiretroviral therapy and its correlation with survival rates.* This development underscores the importance of providers keeping pace with the latest research and clinical findings.
>
> *Source: Kitahata, M.M., Gange, S.J., Abraham, A.G., Merriman, B., Saag, M.S., Justice, A.C., Moore, R.D. (2009, April 30). Effect of early versus deferred antiretroviral therapy for HIV on survival. *New England Journal of Medicine, 360(18)*, 1815-26.

Notwithstanding a number of training programs across the country, some participants discussed their interactions with providers who seemed not to have stayed abreast of HIV care and treatment issues.

To address this, the American Academy of HIV Medicine suggested, "Rotations in HIV care and/or exposure to populations impacted by HIV should be expanded…along with outpatient opportunities for internal medicine and family medicine residence." They added that "clinical training opportunities, satellite learning, and consultation through teleconferences and Web-based programs should be expanded and encouraged for primary care providers already in the field."

Respondents also emphasized the need for health professionals to undergo cultural competency training so they understand not only what but whom they are treating. Since the onset of the epidemic, this has been an enormous concern for gay and bisexual men, who were initially simply ignored by many health professionals. The transgender community continues to note significant levels of discrimination from a medical community that may not understand them or their needs. Cultural competency extends beyond the issue of sexual orientation or gender identification, however, to include, age, substance use, and race/ethnicity. For example, "Native peoples have distinct and unique approaches to health and wellness, based upon their respective cultural values and traditions," said one New York City resident. "Socio-cultural and individual factors contribute to the growing HIV problem among Asian and Pacific Islanders," added a Brooklyn, New York native.

E. Summary

Improving access to care and enhancing health outcomes for underserved people living with HIV can be a complex undertaking. Access to HIV/AIDS health care can often be facilitated for those lacking private health insurance through an array of public programs. However, the need for HIV/AIDS care is often just one of many needs, especially for those living in poverty and with social problems that often accompany HIV/AIDS. Left unaddressed, these nonmedical needs can affect how people access care, and, ultimately, health outcomes.

At community forums and in written submissions, individuals explored the multitude of factors that must be addressed if access to care and improved health is to become a reality for all people. Certainly, access to HIV/AIDS care is important, particularly access to care for related conditions and essential social services, like housing, transportation, and job training.

Ultimately, the particular services that are needed differ for each person, and comments conveyed that providers serving people living with HIV must recognize each individual's unique needs and circumstances. One San Francisco doctor succinctly described the issue: "Treating HIV/AIDS is not a one-size-fits-all situation."

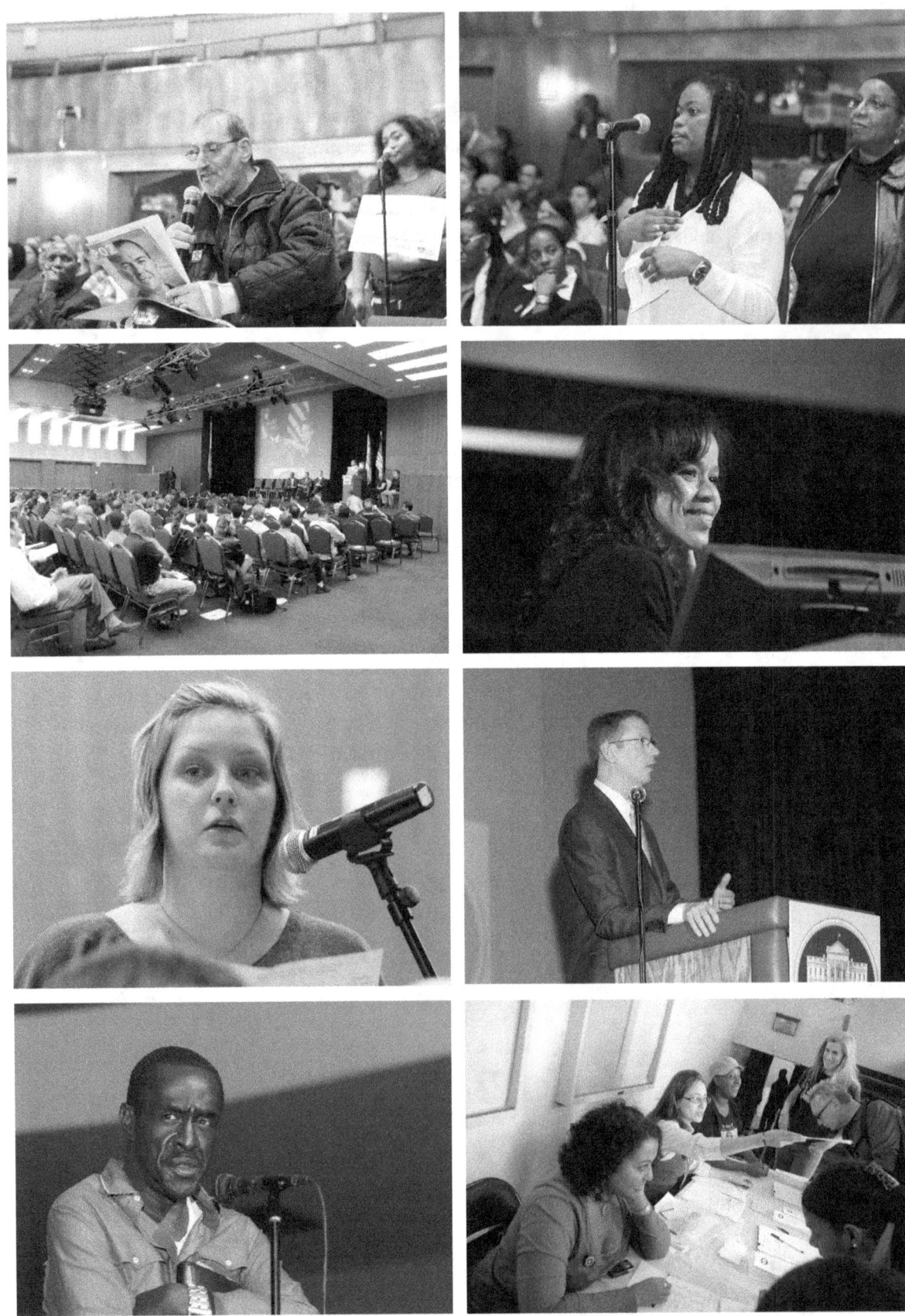

Reducing HIV-Related Health Disparities

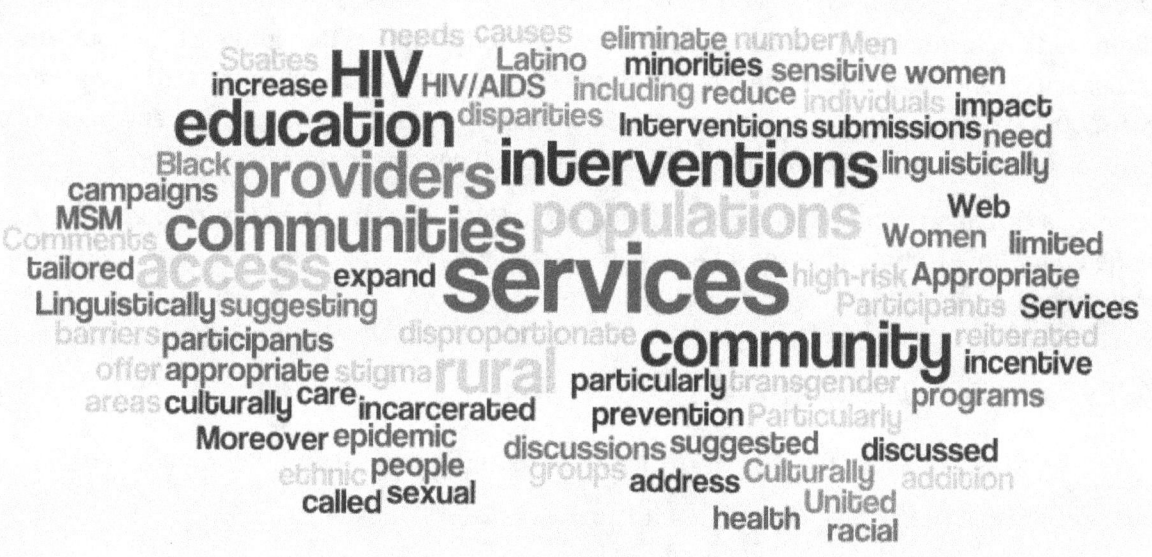

HIV has had a disproportionate impact on specific populations, since the beginning of the HIV epidemic. Three quarters of HIV/AIDS diagnoses are among men in the United States, and men who have sex with men are particularly impacted by the epidemic. Approximately one-half of all persons living with HIV in the United States are MSM, and MSM account for 53 percent of new HIV infections each year.[80] CDC scientists have determined that MSM are 44 to 86 times more likely to become infected with HIV than other men and 40 to 77 times more likely to become infected than women.[81] Moreover, MSM is the only risk group in the United States whose estimated annual number of new infections is increasing. A disproportionate number of HIV diagnoses among MSM are MSM of color. Communities of color, especially the African-American and Latino communities, are also disproportionately impacted by HIV. For example:

- Approximately 71 percent of all HIV/AIDS cases diagnosed in 2007 were among racial and ethnic minorities.[82]

- While comprising just 13 percent of the U.S. population, African-Americans accounted for 47 percent of the estimated AIDS cases diagnosed in 2007; Latinos make up 15.4 percent of the population, yet comprise 17 percent of AIDS cases.[83,84]

---

80. CDC. (2009, August). *HIV and AIDS among gay and bisexual men.* Retrieved from the CDC Web site: http://www.cdc.gov/NCHHSTP/newsroom/docs/FastFacts-MSM-FINAL508COMP.pdf., p. 1.

81. .CDC. (2010), *CDC Analysis Provides New Look at Disproportionate Impact of HIV and Syphilis Among U.S. Gay and Bisexual Men.* Retrieved from the CDC Web site: http://www.cdc.gov/nchhstp/Newsroom/msmpressrelease.html

82. CDC. (2009, August). *HIV/AIDS among African Americans.* Retrieved from the CDC Web site: http://www.cdc.gov/hiv/topics/aa/resources/factsheets/pdf/aa.pdf., p. 1.

83. U.S. Census Bureau. (2008). *State and county quick facts: USA.* Retrieved from the Census Bureau Web site: http://quickfacts.census.gov/qfd/states/00000.html.

84. CDC. (2009). *HIV/AIDS surveillance report, 2007, 19,* 1.

- Although women account for a quarter of HIV/AIDS cases in the United States, 84 percent of HIV/AIDS cases among women are among women of color, with African-American women accounting for more than three of every five cases.[85]

Disparities are also evident in the geographic distribution of HIV/AIDS cases in the United States with a disproportionate number of HIV cases occurring in the South as well as the Northeast. Although over 80 percent of reported AIDS cases in the United States between 1994 and 2007 occurred in large (more than 500,000 persons) metropolitan areas, the South has the largest number and percentage of AIDS cases diagnosed in nonmetropolitan areas (less than 50,000 persons) in the United States.

People participating in our national conversation about HIV/AIDS underlined that resources must be targeted to those communities most heavily affected by the epidemic. They offered specific recommendations for action:

A. Expand Services to At-Risk Populations

"[We need] to ensure that communities with small populations have access to resources, and to develop strategies for emerging communities."

—New York City, New York community discussion

Racial and Ethnic Minorities

The call for swift action to address health disparities among racial and ethnic minorities was an overarching theme throughout the community discussions and in the many submissions made to ONAP.

As the National Medical Association wrote in its submission to ONAP, "Persons of color living with HIV/AIDS are more likely to experience a myriad of social and economic challenges that inevitably exacerbate the conditions known to be associated with this disease." They added, "The negative impact of HIV infection will become increasingly salient over time."

Policy Recommendation to Address HIV Disease Among Black Americans

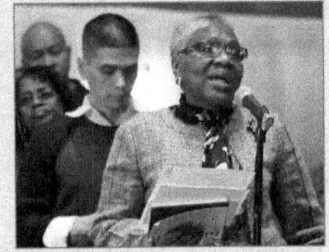

Across several community discussions and Web submissions, individuals expressed a need for policy makers to speak with stakeholders from communities of color. In particular, many people asked for a more focused response targeting the African-American community. They asked that the National HIV/AIDS Strategy include provisions for funding grants and initiatives in the African-American community and create periodic reports on the work being done and the outcomes achieved.

---

85. CDC. (2009). *HIV/AIDS surveillance report, 2007, 19, 1, 17.*

Given the disproportionate burden of HIV among African-Americans, many people advocated for a declaration of a national state of emergency regarding HIV/AIDS in the African-American community. In San Francisco, we heard this plea:

> "African-Americans have been disproportionately affected by HIV/AIDS since the epidemic's beginning and that disparity has deepened over time…we must do something about it. I would like to ask you to please consider recommending, implementing, and declaring a national state of emergency within the African-American community and allocating resources accordingly."

Significant public attention was given to other racial and ethnic minority groups as well. A number of individuals, particularly at the New York City and Minneapolis meetings, discussed the unique challenges faced by African immigrants. Discussions also emphasized the particular needs of Asian/Pacific Islanders, Native Americans, and Latinos.

Latinos are the fastest growing minority group in the Nation. As of 2008, Latinos continue to represent a growing proportion of HIV cases. Nearly one out of five HIV/AIDS cases diagnosed in the United States in 2007 were among this population.[86] Puerto Rico was among the top 10 States and Territories in terms of AIDS cases in 2007.[87]

Health Disparities Among Racial/Ethnic Minorities Living With HIV/AIDS

- Immigrants are more likely than native-born U.S. residents to present for care with an AIDS-defining illness.

- African-Americans accounted for approximately 49 percent of new HIV infections diagnosed in 2007. African-Americans suffer disproportionate rates of diabetes, heart disease, and stroke and are more likely than their White counterparts to die from cancer.

- Racial/ethnic minorities in care are less likely than their White counterparts to be taking antiretroviral therapy.

Sources: Weiwel E, Nasrallah H, Hannah D, et al. *HIV diagnosis and care initiation among foreign-born persons in New York City, 2001-2007.* Presentation at the 16th Conference on Retroviruses and Opportunistic Infections; February 8-11, 2009; Montreal, Quebec.

CDC HIV/AIDS Surveillance Report. 2007; 19. Table 1.

U.S. Department of Health and Human Services, Office of Minority Health. African American profile. n.d. Available at: http://minorityhealth.hhs.gov/templates/browse.aspx?lvl=2&lvlID=51. Accessed December 15, 2009.

Stone VE. Physician contributions to disparities in HIV/AIDS care: the role of provider perception regarding adherence. *Curr HIV/AIDS Rep.* 2005 Nov; 2(4): 189-93.

---

86. CDC. (2009, August). *HIV/AIDS among Hispanics/Latinos.* Retrieved from the CDC Web site: http://www.cdc.gov/hiv/hispanics/resources/factsheets/hispanic.htm.

87. CDC. (2007). *Basic statistics.* Retrieved from the CDC Web site: http://www.cdc.gov/hiv/topics/surveillance/basic.htm.

"Negative cultural influences and stigma are big challenges for [Latinos], and we need interventions that will address core family values among the Hispanic community as well as traditionalism and machismo," said a Laredo, Texas Health Department employee. Many participants added stigma to the list of barriers impeding HIV testing and care within the Latino population.

One common suggestion for improving health disparities, particularly among Blacks and Latinos, was to involve religious leaders and faith-based organizations. "Religiosity plays an important role in the life of most Hispanics or Latinos. It is estimated that 75 percent of Latinos arriving in the United States consider themselves Catholic," explained a Miami, Florida community participant. She added, "In our experience, for the majority of Latinos—no matter their country of origin or whether recently arrived or living in the United States for many years—the church represents a safe, nonthreatening place to go for services beyond spiritual counseling."

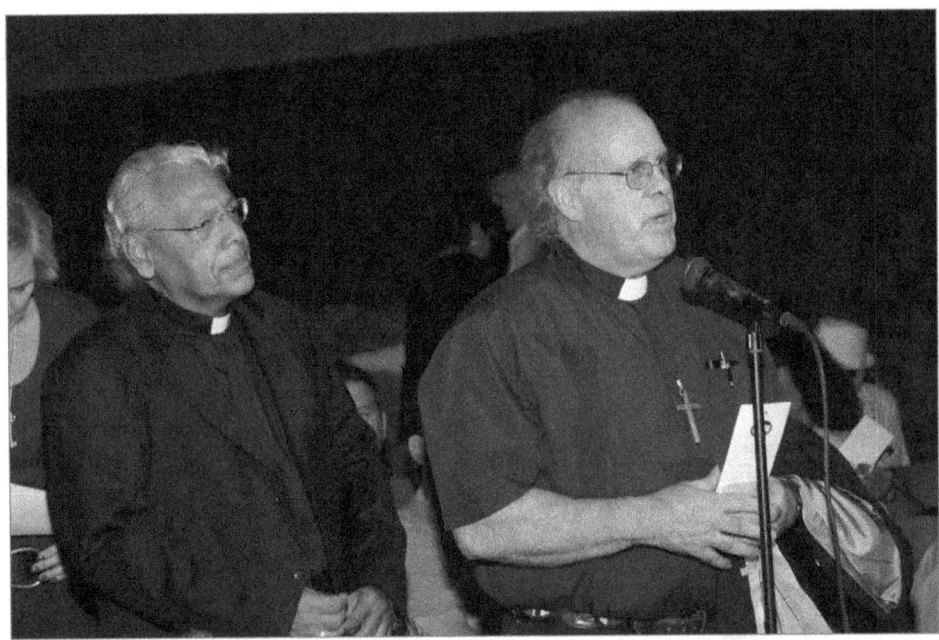

Recognizing spirituality as well as traditional health practices were highlighted as important aspects of culturally competent care for a range of racial and ethnic minorities. As a New York community discussion respondent suggested, "Support the integration of traditional health care practices, which includes the use of traditional medicine practitioners within the HIV/AIDS service delivery system…for Native Americans."

American Indian/Alaska Native advocates and consumers expressed concern that misperceptions about their community were a cause of health disparities. They noted that many Native Americans live in urban areas, not just on reservations, and they highlighted the diversity of tribes and cultures.[88,89] Participants asserted that such diversity should be considered when devising prevention and care strategies.

---

88. Office of Minority Health. (2009, October 21). American Indian/Alaska Native profile. Retrieved from the Minority Health Web site: http://minorityhealth.hhs.gov/templates/browse.aspx?lvl=2&lvlID=52.

89. HRSA. (2008, August). *American Indians, Alaska Natives, and HIV/AIDS*. Retrieved from the HRSA Web site: ftp://ftp.hrsa.gov/hab/Native.Amer.pdf., p. 1.

One person suggested consulting with the 13 U.S. Indigenous Epidemiology Centers to create a broader, more tailored approach. Similar sentiments were echoed by a Ohio man: "Prevention messages must be available in multiple Asian languages (including over 100 languages), and be culturally sensitive."

Women

"The face of HIV is changing and [we] need to be target[ing] women," explained a Jackson, Mississippi resident. Women represent 26 percent of HIV/AIDS cases diagnosed in 2007, of which 83 percent were attributed to heterosexual contact.[90] "A heterosexual woman's biggest infector is a man, whether that man is heterosexual, gay, down low or in prison," wrote a woman from Pennsylvania. "I am not HIV-positive," wrote a woman from Florida, "but I have been myself a woman at risk. I have lost friends and co-workers because of HIV/AIDS, and for the past eleven (11) years I have shared my life with my husband, who now has AIDS." ONAP heard from numerous women living with HIV who were infected by their male partners. As a woman from Kansas explains,

"I was very much like so many people ... I thought that AIDS did not affect me. I am a college educated African American Female who had been married for 15 years with 3 small children when I began this unexpected journey and received an HIV+ diagnosis. Of course I had no risk factors, I knew my risk but I did not know my husband's risk."

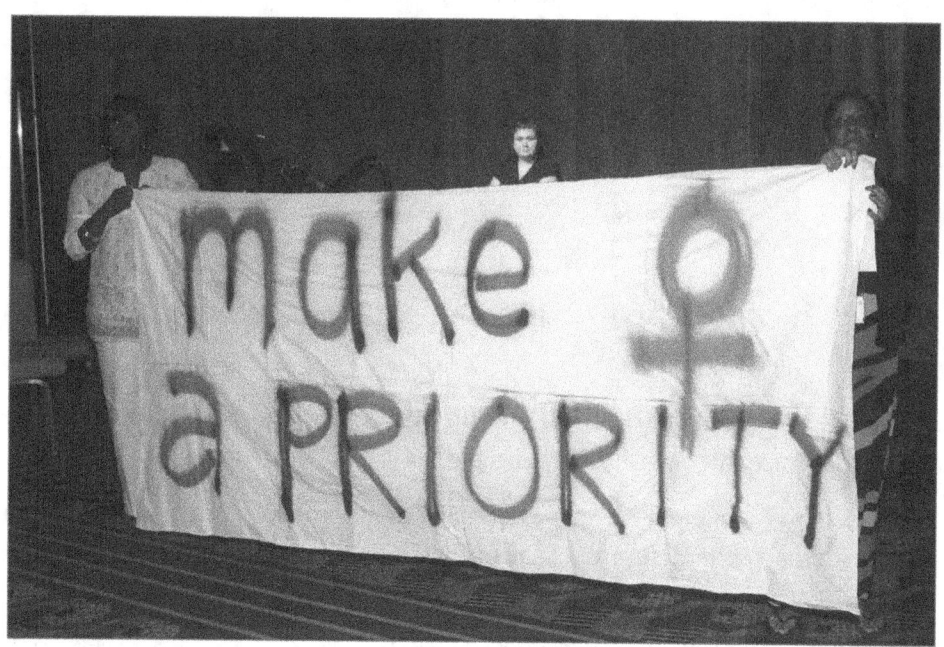

---

90. CDC. (2009, August). *HIV/AIDS in the United States.* Retrieved from the CDC Web site: http://www.cdc.gov/hiv/resources/factsheets/PDF/us.pdf., p. 1.

Among women, there are diverse sets of challenges. For some women living with HIV, the responsibilities of care giving, or working two jobs, is the primary impediment to ongoing health care. Among others, trauma, violence, and stigma inhibit health care seeking behaviors and give rise to comorbidities associated with HIV/AIDS. As one participant explained, "We learned that a lot of these females have dual diagnoses. They are substance users. They have mental health issues and a lot of them are in treatment facilities…and they are not knowledgeable of the disease."

Participants cited gender-based inequities, underestimated HIV risk, and lower socioeconomic levels as some of the issues undercutting women's ability to access appropriate health care.

Participants advocated for peer-based approaches in outreach, messaging, and service delivery targeting women. "Actively recruit and fund more communal, cultural, homegrown interventions by women of color for women of color," said a Houston, Texas woman. "When we train women to be peer educators, they exhibit a lot more ownership of the prevention messages that we teach them and they often adopt them in their own lives and then go on to adopt safer behavior [and] communicate [that] to their communities," added an Albuquerque, New Mexico woman.

Men who have sex with men

Several recommendations reflected concern over Federal policies that discouraged health promotion activities that target gay and bisexual men and the de-emphasis of men who have sex with men overall as a priority population for HIV-prevention activities. One Washington, D.C. resident commented:

"I am particularly speaking from the standpoint of a gay man here this evening, one who has lived with HIV for 27 years, that first and foremost in the legislative agenda we need to end the restrictive provisions of Section 2500 Public Health Service Act. It is ridiculous that we cannot have frank, adequate, explicit education aimed at our communities. [And] rolled up within that is the inadequacy of CDC interventions aimed at gay and bisexual men… at this time only 4 of 17 of the approved interventions target us, but yet we represent over half of the new HIV infections."

Other comments pointed to the diversity among MSM populations and the need for prevention responses that recognize this diversity. For example:

- Some MSM may culturally identify as bisexual or heterosexual and not respond to messaging or care approaches targeting "out" gay men.
- The influence of culture on HIV risk should be recognized. Culture can be a protective factor. Among Latino MSM, greater acculturation into U.S. culture has been associated with increased risk behaviors for HIV infection.[91,92]

---

91. Marks, G, (1998). Is acculturation associated with sexual risk behaviours? An investigation of HIV-positive Latino men and women. *AIDS Care, 10,* 283 295.

92. Rojas-Guyler, L,, Ellis, N,, & Sanders, S. (2005). Acculturation, health protective sexual communication, and HIV/AIDS risk behavior among Hispanic/Latino women in a large midwestern city. *Health Education & Behavior, 32,767,* 779.

- A greater proportion of Black and Latino MSM become infected with HIV between ages 13 and 29 than do White MSM.[93]

- Noninjection drug use is associated with HIV risk behavior and HIV infection among MSM, but substance use patterns differ markedly across MSM by race and ethnicity, and geography.[94]

Many participants called for increased prevention education and more targeted efforts, including tapping into online social and dating venues for risk reduction messages, and utilizing positive role models to reach various segments of MSM. A great deal of public attention was given to young MSM. In a written submission, the Gay Men's Health Crisis called for:

"School interventions that promote tolerance and acceptance of LGBT [lesbian, gay, bisexual, transgender] youth. Gay/straight alliances and anti-bullying curricula correlate with lower HIV risk behavior… and better health and school performance outcomes. HHS and CDC should [also] promote parental acceptance as a public health imperative."

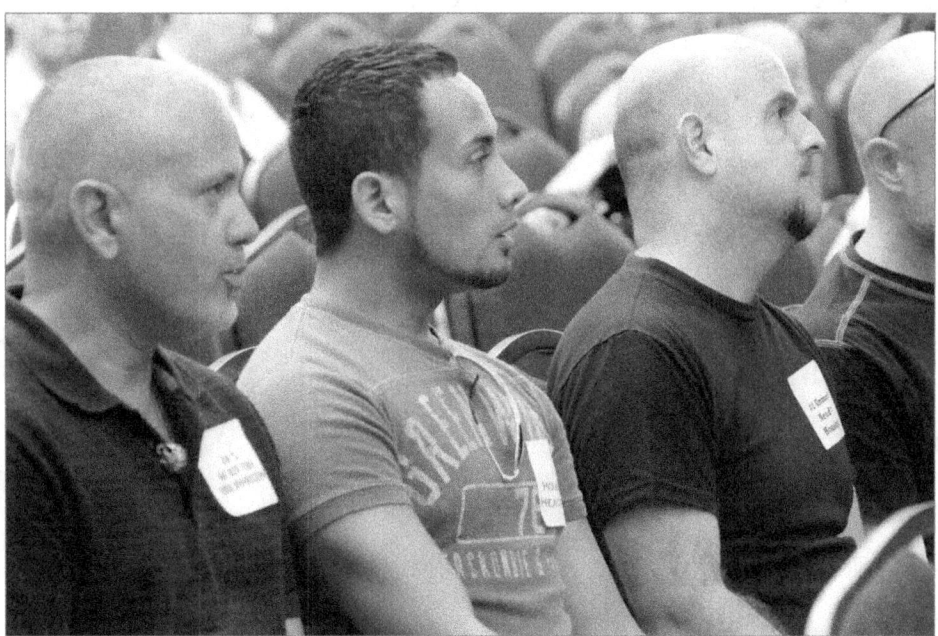

Transgender Persons

Many participants stated that transgender populations have been overlooked by HIV prevention programs. The Los Angeles County HIV Prevention Planning Committee Transgender Task Force stated that, "The transgender population, while estimated to be relatively small compared to other populations, is disproportionately affected by HIV, and has among the highest seroprevalence rates of any group."

---

93. CDC. (2009, August). *HIV and AIDS among gay and bisexual men*. Retrieved from the CDC Web site: http://www.cdc.gov/NCHHSTP/newsroom/docs/FastFacts-MSM-FINAL508COMP.pdf., p. 2.

94. CDC. CDC fact sheet: HIV and AIDS among gay and bisexual men. August 2009. Available at: http://www.cdc.gov/NCHHSTP/newsroom/docs/FastFacts-MSM-FINAL508COMP.pdf. Accessed January 29, 2010.

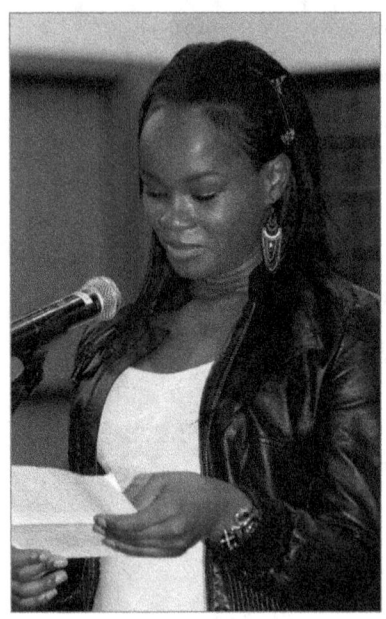

According to a recently published CDC study, estimates of HIV/AIDS prevalence among transgender populations are as high as 27 percent.[95] Other reports have documented that transgender individuals experience higher rates of abuse and institutional discrimination;[96] face unique legal challenges (e.g. qualifying for services where identification and current name do not match);[97] and may be more susceptible to HIV from survival sex or injection practices associated with hormonal therapies or silicone.[98]

Participants called for increased inclusion of transgender individuals in clinical trials and research. They asked that HIV and other health information be crafted and distributed to reach transgender individuals. Respondents also highlighted the need to better educate the public and health professions to ensure transgender individuals can receive culturally-competent care. These sentiments are summed up by a Web submission from Virginia:

"[Government agencies] have continually neglected to include transgender populations in the ways that they capture data about HIV prevalence and incidence, in the prevention interventions that they promote for health departments and community based organizations that they fund, and in making the care services accessible for HIV positive transgender persons. This is not to say that no progress has occurred, but especially considering the extremely high levels of infection among some urban transgender communities, it is clear that more needs to be done urgently."

---

95. Herbst, J.H., Jabocs, E.D., Finlayson, T.J., McKleroy, V.S., Neumann, M.S., & Crepaz, N. (2008). Estimating HIV prevalence and risk behaviors of transgender persons in the United States: a systematic review. *AIDS and Behavior, 12(1)*, 1–17.

96. HRSA. (2009, September). *HRSACareAction: Intimate Partner Violence.* Retrieved from the HRSA Web site: http://hab.hrsa.gov/publications/september2009/September2009.pdf., p. 4.

97. Ibid., p. 4.

98. Xavier, J., Honnold J.A., & Bradford, J. (2007). The health, health-related needs, and lifecourse experiences of transgender Virginians. *Community Health Research Initiative Center for Public Policy, Virginia Commonwealth University and Virginia HIV Community Planning Committee and Virginia Department of Health.*

Incarcerated Populations

Each year about one in four people living with HIV spend time in a correctional facility.[99] Some of the same socioeconomic and psychosocial factors associated with increased risk for HIV infection are also associated with incarceration. These include homelessness, poverty, substance use, and lack private insurance coverage.[100,101,102,103,104]

In the United States, Blacks and Latinos are more likely to be incarcerated than other racial or ethnic groups. Since Blacks and Latinos accounted for 63 percent of incarcerated individuals in 2002, interventions and investment specifically targeting these populations are needed.[105]

Across community discussions, individuals discussed the need to prevent both HIV and incarceration, better treat those already incarcerated, and improve re-entry programs to ensure HIV-positive individuals are connected to the services they need.

"We need…continuity of care for individuals leaving corrections facilities," said an Arkansas man. "Increas[e] health care linkages from prison," said a Pennsylvania resident. Or as a Web respondent expressed, "When patients are released, they should be given two weeks to 30-day supply of medications and community resource/provider information to schedule an appointment. Often patients are released without or with only a few days' supply of medication, and no linkage to health care." A respondent from Virginia elaborated on this point and the consequences of interrupted treatment:

"Because of medication/drug resistance, you cannot stop and start HIV medication as people do with diabetes, cholesterol and blood pressure treatment. Lack of treatment, delayed treatment, and treatment interruption, negatively impact an HIV-infected person's health status and can limit their treatment options in the future. The result is greater costs incurred in the medical care of an infected person who is less well than someone who had consistent access to treatment and health care."

---

99. Okie, S. (2007, January 11). Sex, drugs, prisons, and HIV. *New England Journal of Medicine, 356(2),* 106.

100. Cho, Richard, Corporation for Supportive Housing. (2008, March). Overlap and Interaction of Homelessness and Incarceration: A Review of Research and Practice. NAHC Research Summit.

101. National Health Care for the Homeless Council. (2008). *Incarceration, homelessness, and health.* Retrieved from the NHCHC Web site: http://www.nhchc.org/Advocacy/PolicyPapers/Incarceration2008.pdf.

102. National Mental Health Association. (2007). *Position statement 52: In support of maximum diversion of persons with serious mental illness from the criminal justice system.* Retrieved from: http://www.mentalhealthamerica.net/go/position-statements/52.

103. CDC. (2009). *HIV/AIDS surveillance report, 2007,* 19, Table 3.

104. HRSA. (2008). *The power of connections.* Retrieved from the HRSA Web site: http://hab.hrsa.gov/publications/progressreport08/2008ProgressReport.pdf., p. 25.

105. Human Rights Watch. (2002, February). *Race and incarceration in the United States.* Retrieved from the Human Rights Watch Web site: http://www.hrw.org/legacy/backgrounder/use/race.

B. Provide Culturally and Linguistically Appropriate Services and Interventions

"We should start looking [at] individuals, their cultures, and what the underlying needs are."

—Brooklyn, New York Web submission

Many participants at the community discussions spoke emphatically about the importance of culturally and linguistically appropriate services for people living with HIV.

A New York City man recommended messages be developed that are "specific to individual ethnic populations in their language and/or culture." A California resident explained,

"L.A. County sprawl[s] over 4,800 square miles. We come from diverse cultures and ethnicities. We speak many languages. We are Asian/Pacific Islander, Middle Eastern, African-American; we are White, and yes we are Latino. Los Angeles is home to the largest population of Mexicanos outside of Mexico City. It has the highest concentration of people from El Salvador than any other place in this Nation. We have many unique differences and many unique needs when it comes to HIV and AIDS."

Many people told us that greater funding and more interventions targeting sexual and racial and ethnic minorities are needed. Participants noted the importance of utilizing minority-run, community-based organizations to help remove barriers associated with distrust of the health system, misinformation, stigma, and immigration status. Participants also discussed cash-strapped organizations that struggle to survive. Participants at the community forums emphasized using minority-run organizations to reduce cultural insensitivity or compromised health care. According to one organization, "[W]e found that in primary care, 30 percent of transgender people do not go to see health care [providers] because of discrimination and disrespect that they have had in the past." "Target research interventions and funding to underserved populations, including aboriginal groups, linguistic minorities, adolescents, women, active drug users, and persons who come late into HIV care," a Florida man recommended. "We need free, confidential, small, open forums culturally sensitive regardless of immigration status or sexual orientation to address our differences as women and as Latinas," added one Web respondent.

C. Improve Availability of HIV-Related Services in Rural Areas and U.S. Territories

"[HIV/AIDS] is exacerbated by poverty, lower levels of education which are correlated with lack of information about HIV and AIDS, and fewer jobs in rural areas especially for the kinds of jobs that would provide health benefits."
—Columbia, South Carolina community discussion

The need for increased health and social services in rural areas and U.S. Territories is clear:

- Nearly one-half of rural residents suffer from at least one chronic illness;[106]
- Rural residents are more likely to live below the Federal poverty level than their urban counterparts;[107] and
- HIV-positive rural residents are less likely to receive highly active antiretroviral therapy than those in urban areas.[108]

HIV/AIDS care delivery in rural geographic areas is a challenge often because of stigma and a shortage of trained providers willing to treat people living with HIV.

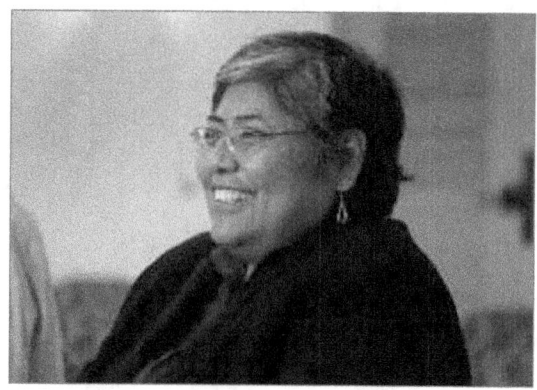

"Most consumers must travel to larger cities for dental services, and even then many dentists don't accept ADAP, or Medicaid. The same is true of mental health services," explained a person living with HIV from upstate New York. "Due to these limitations placed on us, we as rural consumers have not been able to lead normal, productive, healthy lives around and within our communities. We need more providers willing to treat those infected with HIV/AIDS and willing to accept the medical coverage afforded to us."

"In addition, the government must recognize that rural residents average fewer medical appointments than their urban areas and the need for increased technology infrastructure in rural areas including high speed Internet," suggested a Minneapolis, Minnesota participant.

---

106. HHS. (2006). *HHS programs to protect and enhance rural health.* Retrieved from the HHS Web site: http://www.hhs.gov/news/factsheet/rural.html.

107. National Rural Health Association. (n.d.) *What is different about rural health care?* Retrieved from the NRHA Web site: http://www.ruralhealthWeb.org/go/left/about-rural-health/what-s-different-about-rural-health-care/what-s-different-about-rural-health-care.

108. RAND Corporation. (2006) *Research brief: Disparities in care for HIV patients: results of the HCSUS study.* Retrieved from the RAND Web site: http://www.rand.org/pubs/research_briefs/2006/RAND_RB9171.pdf.

Respondents concerned with reducing health disparities in rural areas recommended telemedicine programs and CME conferences that give rural providers an opportunity to discuss best practices. They voiced strong support for loan forgiveness programs as incentives for clinicians in areas with a shortage of health care providers. Participants also supported a national education campaign that would decrease HIV stigma and empower HIV-positive individuals in rural communities.

D. Summary

The HIV/AIDS epidemic has had a disproportionate impact on racial, ethnic, and sexual minorities in the United States. Comments from the community discussions and the Web submissions reiterated the need to expand education and prevention services to these communities to address the causes of the disparities. Particularly high-risk groups including MSM, transgender individuals, women, Black and Latino populations, and incarcerated populations should have access to interventions tailored to each community. Moreover, participants also called for more culturally sensitive and linguistically appropriate services and interventions to eliminate barriers to care. Participants also discussed the needs of people in rural communities who have limited access to health providers, particularly those that offer HIV services. In addition to suggesting incentive programs to increase the number of providers in rural areas, they also suggested education campaigns to reduce HIV stigma.

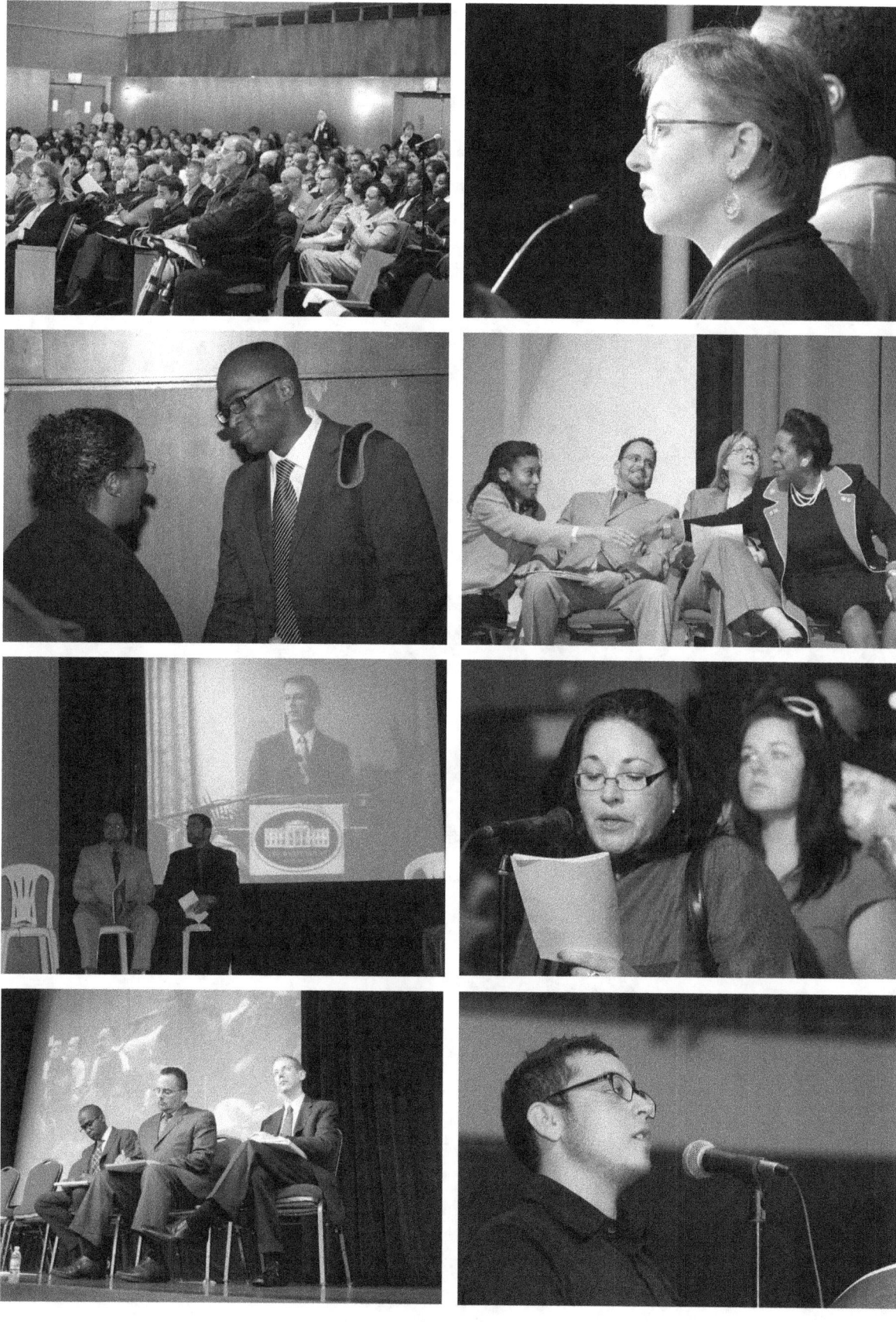

Crosscutting Themes

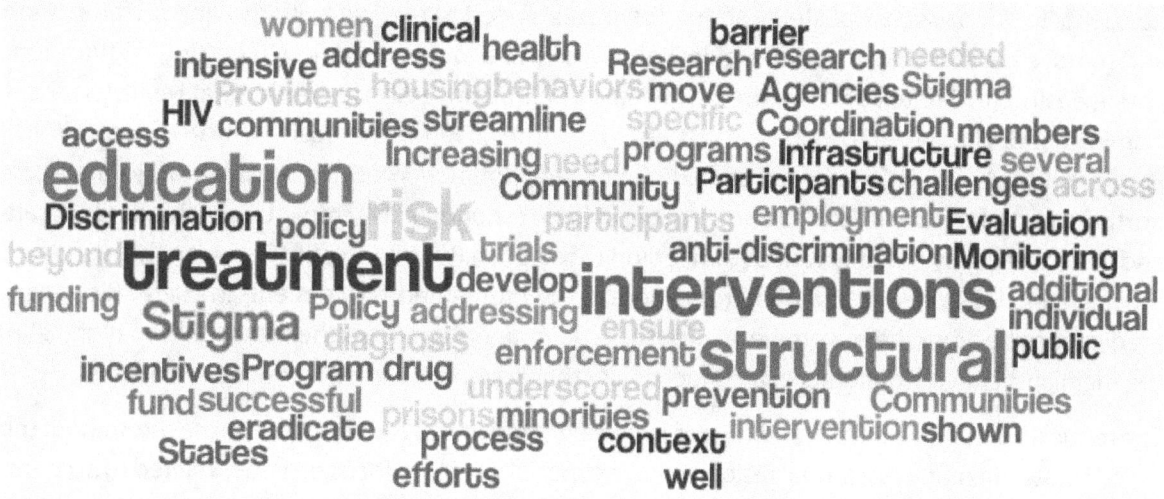

Many of the recommendations received do not fit neatly into one of the three key goals for the strategy, but apply to more than one or relate to crosscutting issues. Key crosscutting recommendations include:

A. Evaluation and Program Monitoring

"[Evaluation] is critical so that all of our interventions and the impact that we have on our communities are measured and sufficiently resourced."

—San Francisco community discussion

Many community discussion attendees underscored the need for tracking program performance and outcomes. "Evaluation is needed to maintain effectiveness," explained one respondent. "There needs to be a monitoring and evaluation framework so that we can be able to look back…and say [if] what we implemented has made any sense," added another.

A number of participants called for government at all levels to be held accountable for using public funds appropriately and assuring high quality public services. "Funded agencies need to be held accountable for ever[y] penny spent," said a Tennessee resident. "A funded agency that has found two new positive cases in five years is not right…If an organization or agency is not [finding] new infections, give the money to someone who is willing to do the job."

While people raised the theme of accountability at a number of community discussions, perhaps nowhere was it stressed more so than in Puerto Rico. Some of the issues related to Puerto Rico may be unique to the island. A common recommendation that we heard in Puerto Rico was for the Federal Government to consider directing funds to a third party administrator instead of sending the funds to the commonwealth government.

"I want to denounce the high level of bureaucracy that corrupts the Health Department," said one community discussion respondent. "This country…has mismanaged the delivery of care and prevention of AIDS and it is time [that] the funds are given [directly] to the agencies that provide the care," said another. Residents in Puerto Rico repeatedly stated there was a need to expedite HIV funding dissemination and remove barriers that impede care delivery. "We have a lot of frustration in getting certifications and licensing [for] detox and treatment…SAMHSA [Substance Abuse and Mental Health Services Administration] has taken so long," said one attendee. "The government receives [Ryan White HIV/AIDS Program] Part A, B, and C but many of those funds [are] not forwarded; it almost [always] stays in the northern part of the Island," stated another Puerto Rico respondent. Discrepancies in standards of care and service capacity not only varied from region to region in Puerto Rico, but between the island and the mainland U.S. A Web respondent from Puerto Rico commented, "HIV patients in Puerto Rico…lack medications because the government imposes requirements to access them that are too high… [In] the mainland, states' requirements are much lower than here. Can somebody explain that?"

The request for more equitable funding and increased standards of care, however, arose throughout the United States. In many cases, rural residents were especially likely to focus on issues related to accountability for public resources. "There needs to be [more] specificity…regarding funding priorities in order [to] address the needs of rural areas because they are different from metropolitan areas. Currently criteria mandates are not sensitive to rural needs," suggested a Jackson, Mississippi resident. But we also heard from people in large metropolitan areas who stressed the importance of evaluating available resources and how those resources are applied. "There is a lot of overlap and as the budget is being constrained [we need] to effectively see what works and what does not work," said a California woman.

B. Coordination Across Agencies, States, Communities, and Providers

"We recommend that the Federal Government review the coordination of funding for HIV/AIDS, substance abuse, and mental health services on the Federal and State level, with the goal of increasing access to these services for patients with HIV."

—Ryan White Medical Providers Coalition submission

On multiple occasions, participants asked for greater coordination among the Federal, State, and local agencies addressing HIV/AIDS. "There are so many different funding [channels] and all of these disparate parts do not work together effectively," explained one public health employee. "There has really got to be a more coordinated effort…because there is just no way for all of us to meet all of the requirements from all of these different departments."

"Federal departments utilize differing income standards, definitions, age groupings, demographic categories, etc.," added another participant. "This causes confusion in matters such as reporting, setting priorities, developing objectives, understanding regulations, [and] evaluating outcomes. It can also make comparisons difficult, if not impossible, between programs."

> **Public Urges More Collaboration Among Federal Agencies**
>
> Greater collaboration can help the Nation better address crosscutting issues ranging from rural health to workforce shortages. Examples of recent collaborations relevant to HIV/AIDS and affected populations include the following:
>
> - CDC and the Department of Health and Human Services Office of Minority Health and the Department of Education have formed the Federal Collaboration on Health Disparities Research.
>
> - The Substance Abuse and Mental Health Services Administration convened a national summit on methamphetamine and included HRSA, CDC, the Office of Women's Health, Indian Health Services, the Office of Minority Health, National Institute on Drug Abuse, and the Department of Justice.

In addition, respondents emphasized coordinating funding applications and reporting mechanisms so providers can streamline administrative tasks and focus attention and resources on more direct services. Some stressed the importance of better collaboration among agencies that may fund similar services to reduce duplication of services and better target financial resources.

Participants also highlighted the importance of coordination among various providers to create a more seamless transition from testing to treatment. As a Los Angeles man explained,

> "I found out that I was HIV positive four blocks from here at the L.A. Gay & Lesbian Center....they took me to a case manager, a social worker, and made appointments for me for crisis counseling, for confirmatory tests, for my doctor, for treatment education, and for the medications thereafter."

Community discussion attendees explained that referrals and partnerships are vital for engagement and retention in care. They added that given the competitive funding environment, however, incentives should be created to better facilitate and improve coordination.

C. Stigma and Discrimination

> "There can be no true progress without stigma reduction. Stigma is still the REAL reason so many don't want to know their status, don't get help, or are afraid to be advocates for their own health."
>
> —Hammond, Indiana Web submission

HIV discrimination and stigma were common topics across community discussions. Many expressed frustration over the pervasiveness of HIV stigma nearly 30 years into the HIV epidemic. Studies have shown that HIV stigma is related to delayed HIV testing and care, as well as disclosure to family and friends. People living with HIV can experience violence, rejection, and even eviction from their homes because of their serostatus, and HIV-positive persons continue to report discrimination in employment and health care settings.[109]

A New York City woman discussed her inability to find a dentist who would treat her because she is HIV positive. A Jackson, Mississippi woman talked about being advised by her provider to have an abortion, merely because she was pregnant and HIV positive. A Florida man complained, "I have been refused treatment…. by medical doctors for my HIV on several counts while covered by private insurance… Imagine a world in which medical doctors do not refuse …life saving services to people with HIV/AIDS. Is that too much to ask?"

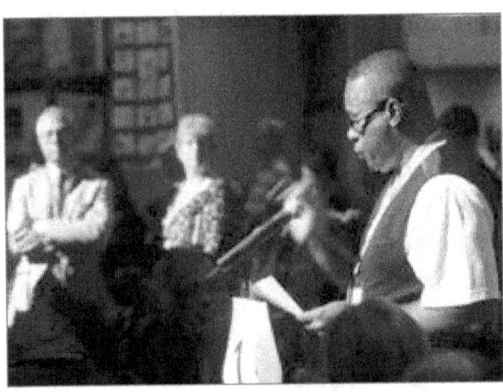

A few community discussion participants simply asked for existing anti-discriminatory policies to be enforced. For instance, the Federal AIDS Policy Partnership suggested, "Issue an Executive Order that requires all Federal agencies [and their contractors] comply with the Rehabilitation Act by barring them specifically from using HIV infection as a basis for categorical exclusion." Participants also discussed the importance of adhering to the Health Insurance Portability and Accountability Act (HIPAA) Privacy Rule to protect personal health information. "Congress should establish stricter penalties for violating HIPAA protections that result in loss of employment, health care coverage, or breech of privacy," stated a New York organization. Enforcement of the Americans with Disabilities Act was similarly highlighted. A San Francisco man who is deaf defended his civil rights under the Americans with Disabilities Act to have access to auxiliary aids and services for effective communication. "I go to school," he noted, "[but the] school does not provide interpreters. When I go to work, they do not provide interpreting service. It is hard to get an interpreter, but we really need it for medical care to be able to speak, to go to a hospital, to get medical needs met."

Discrimination against sexual minorities was mentioned in several community discussions. We heard from those who expressed frustration over the lack of recognition of same sex relationships in visitation policies or insurance coverage.

The commonality across each of these comments is that stigma and discrimination continue to pose significant barriers to those infected or affected by HIV, and the NHAS must address these issues to be successful.

---

109. Herek, G.M., Capitanio, J.P., Widaman, K.F. (2002). HIV-related stigma and knowledge in the United States: prevalence and trends, 1991-1999. *American Journal of Public Health, 92(3)*, 371.

D. Policy

"There is no public policy for screening and testing youth for HIV on the island."
—Puerto Rico community discussion

ONAP received numerous recommendations related to policies that covered a range of issues. Each of these issues is briefly summarized below.

Increasing Infrastructure

Many underscored the need for policies that would address infrastructure gaps in health care and social-service systems, as well as transportation, technology, and housing. Participants called for a policy promoting greater public investment to implement widespread adoption of health information technology. As one submission advocated, portable personal electronic health records have "the ability to transport the detailed record of medical history, drug regimens, and other treatment. They are invaluable for patients with HIV facing relocation, travel, medical emergency, and incarceration….and for [mobile patients] who move from clinic to clinic or State to State."

The challenges associated with rural areas were highlighted by many respondents, especially participants at the South Carolina, Mississippi, and New Mexico meetings. Rural residents advocated for greater investment in social services infrastructure, greater capacity to address HIV at the local level, and more transportation assistance to medical visits.

"[If you live in] the rural areas in the north part of Mississippi, you all have to drive all the way to Tennessee just to get medical care. We need help. We need transportation. We need doctors," one woman exclaimed. "How do you put sufficient infrastructure in funding so that you can maintain a minimum level of services in rural areas?" another participant asked. "It requires a model of funding other than just per capita funding because then your rural areas are always disproportionately on the losing end."

Working with Policy Makers

Many participants in community discussions stressed the importance of dialogue with policy makers because public policy must be informed by the lives and circumstances of people living with HIV. "Our senators and congressmen are responsible for making decisions regarding funding that affects the lives of those of us living with the virus, yet have no idea what living with HIV/AIDS is like," wrote a New Orleans man. "I am concerned that without this knowledge, the decisions are being made based solely on financial numbers and not on the needs of the people receiving the services."

Incentives

Participants also urged that incentives be provided to pharmaceutical companies to further invest in a vaccine, better treatments, or a cure. As one Washington, D.C. man said, "Push the foundations, especially those foundations giving money internationally, to do that here locally and nationally since we are having an economic struggle."

One of the most commonly expressed incentives were policies and programs to encourage recruitment to HIV-related health professions. "Within the past several years, we have seen an exodus of HIV-treating clinicians from the field of HIV medicine," noted a Washington, D.C. physician. "There is also a growing number of clinicians who must spend the majority of their time in non-HIV care in order to support their HIV/AIDS practices, or who take on work and stop seeing these patients altogether."

E. Research

"I have been living with HIV for at least 24 years and I am alive because of research."

—San Francisco, California community discussion

The presence of long-term HIV survivors at community discussions across the country is testament to the power and possibility of research. "I was born HIV positive. I am now 25 years old," said an Elizabeth Glaser Pediatric AIDS Foundation ambassador. "I work full time. I have a great boyfriend and am looking to go on to graduate school." Stories like this illustrate the promise of HIV medications and the role research has played in improving the lives of HIV-positive people. Individuals reminded ONAP that there is still much to do, research questions to explore, and still so much we don't know.

"What are the long-term effects of ARV [antiretroviral] treatment?" asked one respondent. "Why [are] some PLWHA long-term survivors and others suffer increased morbidity and mortality?" asked another. To be able to answer these questions, and to be equipped to address them, participants called for increased investment in research. "Invest more money and meaningful resources in medical and clinical research," said a San Antonio, Texas man.

Community members also noted that more intensive efforts are needed to ensure that women and minorities have access to clinical trials, as well as calls for intervention additional research for specific communities. On several occasions, participants underscored the need to develop and fund structural interventions that address the context of risk and move beyond individual risk behaviors. Participants noted that structural interventions such as education, employment, housing, and drug treatment programs in prisons have been shown to be successful in addressing other public health challenges[110] and that funding these types of structural factors in future research should be a priority.

---

110. Blankenship, K.M., Bray, S.J, Merson, M.H. (2000). *Structural interventions in public health. AIDS, 14(Supplement 1)*, S11–21.

F. Summary

Participants' recommendations addressed several common themes. Primarily, they called for education and anti-discrimination policy enforcement to eradicate stigma that can be a barrier to HIV prevention, diagnosis, and treatment. Comments suggested that to do this, public policy makers should work with community members and advocates to ensure that policies are based on people's medical needs as well as other service needs such as housing assistance. Participants also recommended that these policy makers streamline funding processes and ensure better coordination among Federal agencies, States, communities, and service providers. This will help make navigating the health care system more manageable for people living with HIV and for organizations applying for grants.

Participants suggested that increased coordination could also help to ensure the accountability of federally-funded organizations and public resources for HIV services. Better evaluation and monitoring of these resources would help guarantee that money allocated for HIV/AIDS is being spent effectively and appropriately.

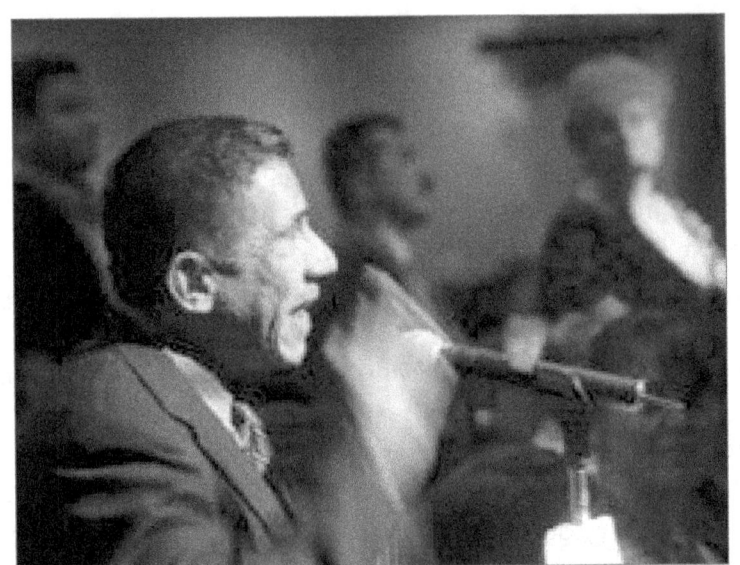
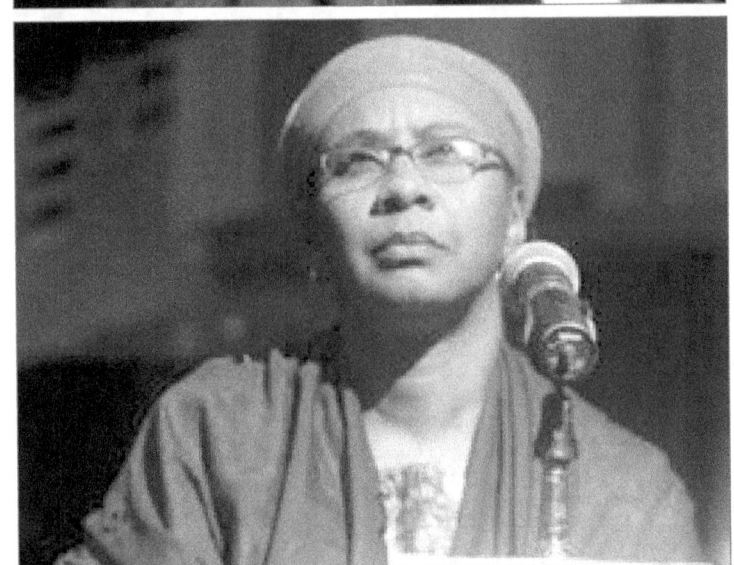
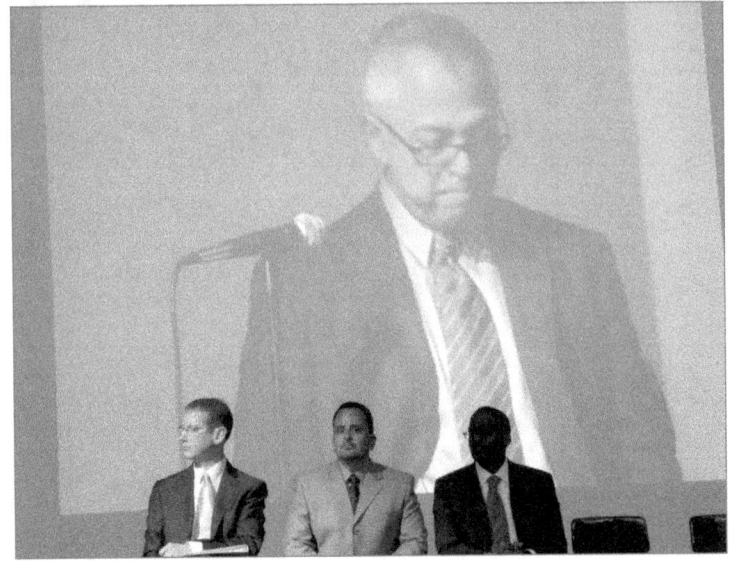

Moving Forward

"Working together, I am confident that we can stop the spread of HIV and ensure that those affected get the care and support they need."
—President Barack Obama

This report will be used to inform the development of a National HIV/AIDS Strategy. The strategy will rely on proven and effective programs and practices.

ONAP has convened a Federal HIV Interagency Working Group—leaders with policy and program expertise in Federal agencies that provide HIV and other related services—to assist with the process of developing the National HIV/AIDS Strategy. The Working Group is tasked with reviewing and prioritizing the many recommendations that ONAP received for the National HIV/AIDS Strategy and analyzing them to identify those actions that hold the most potential for the greatest impact, and for which there is solid scientific evidence of their effectiveness. This report is among several key references that the Working Group will use for developing the strategy.

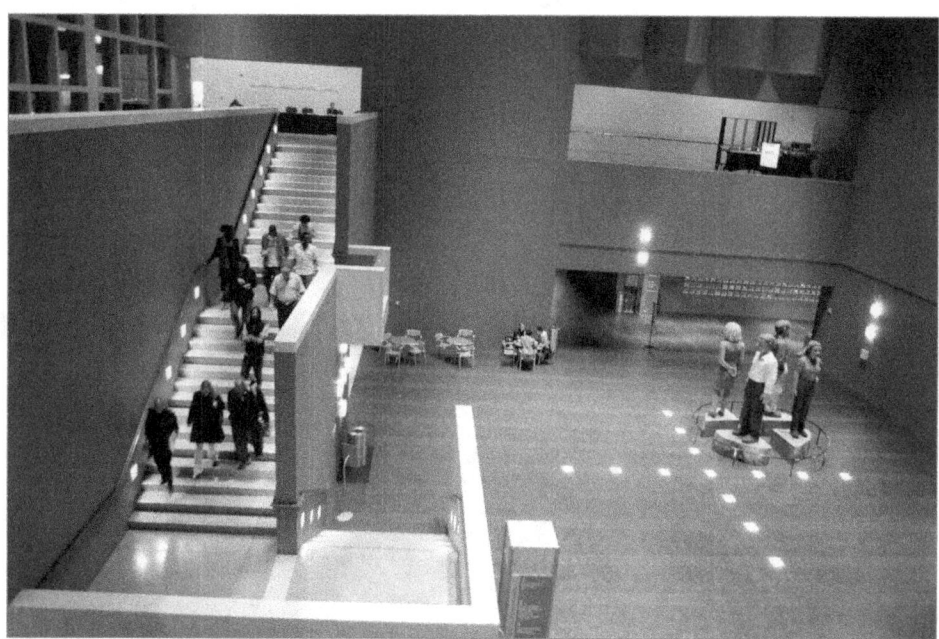

This report aggregates the most common recommendations that ONAP received from the public to provide a mechanism to understand the most commonly held views for the National HIV/AIDS Strategy. In undertaking this effort, the Presidential Advisory Council on HIV/AIDS (PACHA) will have an important role to play in supporting the effective implementation of the strategy and monitoring our progress. This report will be made available to the public via the Web site, http://www.whitehouse.gov/administration/eop/onap/, and will be circulated to the PACHA, as well as Federal agency staff.

Although this report will be among several source materials that will help inform the National HIV/AIDS Strategy, not all topics expressed in this report will be in the final strategy document. As mentioned earlier, the Strategy is not intended to be a comprehensive list of all of the actions, policies, and programmatic priorities needed to respond to the domestic HIV epidemic. Instead, the Strategy will identify a limited number of high payoff steps to address the HIV epidemic in the United States.

In addition to informing the National HIV/AIDS Strategy process, this report may also be a valuable resource for Federal, State, and local agencies, as well as other stakeholders who are working to prevent HIV infection, provide services to people living with HIV, and identify strategies to reduce HIV-related disparities. While not reflecting a scientifically-valid sample of public opinion, this report provides a fairly comprehensive summary of ideas and recommendations from a broad range of interested parties from across the country.

The Office of National AIDS Policy acknowledges and gives sincere thanks to the many individuals who devoted their time and energy to the process by contributing their ideas and sharing their personal stories included in this report.